To Esther Lucile Brown,
with the cordial thanks
of R. ...

The HISTORY

Richard H. Shryock, Ph.D.

WILLIAM H. WELCH PROFESSOR EMERITUS OF
THE HISTORY OF MEDICINE, THE JOHNS HOPKINS UNIVERSITY;
LIBRARIAN OF THE AMERICAN PHILOSOPHICAL SOCIETY

W. B. SAUNDERS COMPANY

PHILADELPHIA & LONDON   1959

# of NURSING

An Interpretation of the

Social and Medical

Factors Involved

4562

Preface

The purpose of this text is not simply to retell the story of nursing. It is, rather, to present that story in close relationship to its scientific as well as to its social background.

The care of the sick has always been influenced by the nature of society at any given time and place—by the type of civilization and by the ideals which were maintained. Nursing in a primitive tribe was obviously different from that in a large city; but it differed also between two urban centers, if one had pagan and the other Christian ideals. Hence, if one is to understand how present nursing emerged, it is necessary to relate it to social history.

More immediately, nursing has always been influenced by the nature of medical practice and by the scientific knowledge available. Nursing in early periods, when not much was known about medicine, could be little more than humane care. But nursing today, when medical science is relatively advanced, is a very different matter. Within the limits of available knowledge, moreover, the role of the nurse has often been conditioned by the role of the physician. It has seemed desirable for these reasons to include medical history in this study, noting for each period how nursing was affected by medical practice, by medical institutions, and by the medical profession.

After all, the modern nurse spends her professional life largely in a medical setting. It is hoped, then, that this study will not only exhibit the influence exerted by medicine on nursing, but will also help to make the present medical environment intelligible in itself. For medicine, like nursing, is illuminated by its past.

v

For some purposes, the recent history of nursing—let us say, since the Nightingale era—is most pertinent for present-day interests. And though an author will wince at the thought, it will be quite possible to pick this book up where one pleases. It seemed best, nevertheless, to begin the narrative at the beginning of Western civilization, in order to attain a vista of the long sweep of nursing through the centuries.

This larger theme may offer, to those who pursue it, some of the values of liberal education. Lest such a statement seem pretentious, let me add that I have in mind chiefly the lift which one experiences in rising above immediate tasks. Important as the latter may be, they take on new significance when fitted into their place in a long and yet unfinished epic.

RICHARD H. SHRYOCK.

Baltimore

Contents

Chapter I

Primitive Medicine and Nursing

Modern medicine, we say, is "scientific"; it deals only with natural phenomena which can be confirmed by all observers. Occult or religious procedures are not employed by the physicians as such, since these do not fall within the province of science as this is now defined. In time of trouble men may appeal to both science and religion, to both the doctor and the priest, but the services of the one are rarely combined with those of the other. There are even persons who turn for help exclusively to science or, conversely, entirely to religion. Thus, men who hold no religious faith depend in illness only on physicians; while such a group as Christian Scientists may leave everything to their religious healers.

Such sharp distinctions, however, are rather recent ones. Vestiges of older outlooks, in which magic, religion, and medicine were indiscriminately combined, survive at the present time. For example, a domestic servant gets a prescription from an out-patient service but then declines to use it except during certain phases of the moon. Here is a trace of astrology—occult lore once cultivated by learned men and still taken seriously in some circles. Or an ignorant midwife emphasizes in her practice the importance of incantations or the provision of certain charms. She puts an axe under the bed in order to "cut labor pains" at the same time that she carries out simple medical procedures. Until very recently much obstetrical practice among southern Negroes was of this nature.

As a matter of fact, magic has not been entirely abandoned even

1

among the educated classes. We now call this "superstition"—a disdainful term—but it has a lingering hold on us. Of course we are also influenced by science and so do not really believe that the number thirteen is unlucky or that we should rap on wood in order to keep the spirits away. Nevertheless, it is so easy to "play safe" in such matters and this does give one a more comfortable feeling. So common is this reaction that some modern hotels still omit "13" in numbering floors. Many would fear to stay on a floor so designated, lest illness or other bad luck ensue. In this situation patrons think they may escape disease by avoiding a mystical number. This is hardly preventive medicine in the modern sense but would have been considered good medicine by most ancient peoples.

Persisting superstitions, then, may help us to understand the outlook of cave-dwelling ancestors. At best, they give only a hint of how early men may have sought to preserve their health. More evidence than this is needed if we are to envisage even the most general aspects of primitive medicine. Just how did such medicine originate and what forms did it take?

Evidence from Archeology and Anthropology

This story is not a simple one. As have all phases of history, medicine and nursing have come down to us through the vast reaches of time. The march of civilization, which used to be viewed as a matter of four or five millennia, is now believed to have been under way for more than a hundred thousand years. Such numbers have little meaning, but it is clear that progress or change of any sort was for most of this time incredibly slow. What went on in human society through all these ages is largely unknown. Only in the last five thousand years have systems of writing been invented, so that we have written records of merely the last small fraction—perhaps of the last fiftieth—of human experience.

It is true that archeologists, digging in the debris beneath ancient villages or scanning the caves where prehistoric peoples once found shelter, can discover something of how these early folk lived and died. Cave men certainly suffered from illness even as we do today, for their bones have been found and show signs of malformation and infection. Even the skeletons of long-extinct animals, for that matter,

2

display lesions of one sort or another. Disease has been the experience of nearly all living things as long as life has existed on earth.

Archeologists also uncover evidence of attempts to find both natural and supernatural remedies. Scattered in ancient graves are objects which apparently were intended to give the wearer magical protection. Also present are bones which show that surgical procedures were occasionally employed, such as placing splints on fractures or trephining skulls. But in the latter case it is not clear whether openings were bored in order to relieve head pains or in order to permit the escape of evil spirits. At any rate, it seems probable that men who operated in this manner also tried other devices against disease. Unfortunately, the evidence about other procedures is usually meager. A skull may reveal something of stone-age surgery but will tell nothing of prehistoric drugs.

What long seemed a more promising way of rediscovering early medicine was suggested by the modern theory of evolution. According to this theory, simple or primitive animal forms persist at the same time that higher forms evolve from them. Thus, we view fishes as an older form of life than are birds or mammals. They represent an early stage of evolution, yet they were at one time the highest type which had yet appeared.

In like manner, in social evolution, human societies were supposed to evolve from simple to complex forms; and modern primitive tribes could be viewed as the surviving representatives of an early stage of this development. If so, the culture of modern savages should reveal a type of civilization through which our ancestors once passed. If we wish to know what the medicine of all peoples was once like, we need only examine that of modern tribes who have never advanced beyond the primitive level. If American Indians used certain charms against disease in 1800, for example, one could assume that similar charms were employed by most peoples when their cultures were in an early stage. What was true of Indians in 1800 must have been true, say, of Europeans in 3,000 B.C.

Anthropologists, however, no longer believe that this was necessarily so. They find that some primitive cultures are quite complex. The marriage customs and secret societies of certain African tribes, for example, are more complicated than our own and have a long history behind them. Their medical procedures also can be intricate

3

and have probably changed with time. And if African medicine of five thousand years ago was different from what it is today, it was no doubt different from that of Europeans in that same remote era.

Tribes have been found, of course, whose culture was cruder than that of most Indians or Africans. The natives of Tasmania, discovered by the Dutch about three centuries ago, used no clothing, knew nothing of bows and arrows, and had never learned to build a hut. Compared to them, the Iroquois Indians possessed a complex civilization. Yet even these Tasmanians had advanced beyond the most primitive stage, for they had developed a language—so essential to all later progress—and knew certain arts such as weaving baskets and the use of fire. Their ways of dealing with sickness may have changed while these skills were being evolved. In a word, the medicine of modern savages is not necessarily the same as was that of prehistoric peoples.

Is there, then, any way of picturing really primitive medicine? Some idea can be formed by examining the earliest records and by observing such elements in the practice of modern primitives as are common to most of them. In both cases there may be vestiges of earlier procedures. One can then reason as intelligently as possible about how these things probably originated. It is known, to begin with, that even animals attempt to relieve pain and to remove the causes of infection. The sick dog turns to grass, apparently for an emetic. The care with which monkeys seemingly remove parasites from each other is one of the attractions of any zoo. A chimpanzee uses its long, black nails to open a sore, very much as human beings do under similar circumstances. It is plausible to assume, then, that simple medical procedures of this sort were pre-human in origin.

The earliest men doubtless did these things instinctively. More intelligent than animals, they must also have tried other devices. Certain of these apparently worked well and were used thereafter, while others seemed ineffective and were discarded. Men thus acquired some medical lore and transmitted it by word of mouth to their descendants.

Here, one may add, was a major difference between men and even the highest animals. The latter, lacking language in the ordinary sense, pass on little learning to their offspring. But man, once he had developed the symbolic sounds called language, taught his children what he had learned from *his* parents and added the results of his own experience. The children thus received most of the knowledge acquired down to their time, and could start where their parents left off in the pursuit of still further information. In a word, knowledge became cumulative. Without this peculiarly human form of behavior, no culture or civilization could have been evolved.

The oldest records indicate that a trial-and-error (empirical) medical lore had long been accumulating among ancient peoples. Egyptian manuscripts, which express the medicine of about 2,000 B.C., for example, reveal much pharmaceutical learning. The Egyptians had evidently tried out hundreds of plant and animal substances during preceding centuries and had recorded those they thought useful as remedies. It is surprising to find what valuable drugs they actually did stumble upon in this way—for example, opium and castor oil.

Again, if one turns to the earliest reports on American Indians, it appears that the Incas of Peru were familiar with the virtues of coca (cocaine) and of cinchona bark (quinine). Other medicaments which are not specific but have some value are found in the earliest lists of various peoples. A study of 144 drugs employed by American Indians shows that no less than 59 of these are still used in modern practice. Here was one reason why European settlers in this country were often favorably impressed by Indian medicine.

On the other hand, many drugs used by primitives had little or no value and some seem outlandish or revolting today. This is indicated by the earliest records, and also by the survival of much nonsense in ancient, medieval, or even modern pharmacopoeias. As late as the American colonial period (1600–1750), our ancestors were consuming such "biologicals" as ground spiders, crab's eyes, lice, worms, and powdered dung. It is really appalling to consider all the materials which have passed down the human alimentary canal in the name of cures! But what was more natural than to assume that, if a patient recovered, whatever had been done for him deserved the credit? And since patients usually did recover, all sorts of things were thereafter assumed to be helpful.

Primitive practice involved more than simple surgery and hit-or-miss drugs. There was undoubtedly a lore about many things that went into or came out of the body. In eating various materials, men inevitably experienced vomiting and purging. Such biologic mecha-

5

nisms had the effect of removing dangerous substances and their operation brought relief. When certain plants were found to set these mechanisms in motion, it seemed sensible to employ them for that purpose. In like manner, early men experienced bleeding, and this—bringing relief in some cases—may also have been practiced artificially. A similarly early origin can be ascribed to certain other medical procedures, such as sweating and bathing in mineral waters. Some of these practices are still routine today, so that we need not be too scornful of remote forebears. Like the cave dweller who discovered the use of fire, the man who first found a good emetic performed a real service to mankind.

Combined with such curative efforts were preventive measures, in so far as prehistoric men found what foods and living habits were conducive to health. It is a striking fact that all modern primitives managed to secure a balanced diet, regardless of what foods are available in different parts of the world. Thus Eskimos, who in winter ate only meat, fared well on this by consuming fats and organic tissues as well as the muscular parts. This may be instinctive; a recent theory holds that even modern children will eat what is good for them if left for any time to their own resources. In any case, what is true here of modern primitives was probably also true of prehistoric man.

Did early man, in addition to finding certain means for preventing or treating illness, go beyond this by seeking out the causes (etiology) of sickness? It is quite likely that, where some natural cause was obvious, he was aware of it and acted accordingly. Trouble following immediately after the bite of a poisonous snake or insect must have been ascribed to these animals, which were thereafter avoided. But most causal factors in disease, as we now know them, were long hidden from view.

The chief advances made by primitives, in what we term medicine, were therefore those empirical treatments and remedies which have just been mentioned. These were found simply by observing natural objects and processes—by learning something about the relations of plants and animals to bodily experience. Here was the beginning of naturalistic medicine of a practical nature. The nearest analogy to it today is folk medicine; that is, the tradition of tried-and-true remedies for simple ills which many families still pass on to their children. This sort of thing could hardly be called science, since no theories or special methods of confirmation were involved. Yet the observation of natural things, even in this simple manner, was the first step toward the development of science as it is now known.

Magic Medicine

Whether there was even a time when men depended entirely on naturalistic or folk medicine of this type, is not clear. This was conceivably the case when the human species first appeared and before anyone had really begun to *think* about health and disease. But wherever actual evidence is found, it is plain that men were already supplementing naturalistic medicine with ideas of an occult nature. Although we now call such ideas superstitious, they were at one time expressions of quite original, creative thought.

Consider, for example, the aforesaid question about the causes of disease. Primitives could detect only the most obvious natural circumstances which led to illness. Yet they had enough imagination to realize that there must be many other causal factors. They also realized that, if these causes could be identified, they might be avoided or overcome in a rational way. It seemed more promising to proceed in this manner than it was just to seek blindly for remedies.

That this was indeed a common attitude is indicated by the historic evidence; all primitives who have been observed think of illness primarily in terms of etiology. Their chief efforts are directed toward uncovering the cause in order to counteract or remove it. But whereas modern medicine demonstrates natural causes, primitive medicine accepted supernatural explanations. We, today, ascribe infections to bacteria; primitives ascribed them to spirits and spells. The logic was the same in both cases, but the nature of the explanation was profoundly different.

Those who take the modern view may naturally inquire: how could uncivilized peoples concoct and believe all this superstitious nonsense? Were stone-age men and modern savages just a stupid lot? The answer is quite the reverse. Belief in the supernatural seems to have resulted from the most intelligent observations which early man could possibly make. This may be illustrated in terms of health and disease, and by the reasoning which primitives probably employed in this connection.

Observations began, as noted, with the identification of certain obvious, natural causes of illness. Men were injured by animals or by one another, and in some of these cases they realized that their sufferings came from external attacks. Evidently, when one experienced pain, there was a cause outside the body. It seemed logical, then, to look for external dangers whenever illness occurred—particularly if this was sudden and serious.

Imagine the reactions of cave men to the sudden collapse of one of their number who had seemed healthy a moment before. It appeared as if he had been struck down by an axe. (We might speak, today, of a cerebral hemorrhage but note that we still call this "a stroke.") Yet there was no evidence of an enemy. This was enormously puzzling to a caveman who knew nothing of physiology—a sort of early detective thriller. Evidently, something unseen had killed the man and in so mysterious a manner that no traces were left behind. There must be dangers lurking about—dangers which could not be seen, heard or sensed in any way. Such things were not natural; that is, they were super-natural. What were these strange influences, why did they strike, and how could one guard against them?

In seeking answers here, primitive thought had to proceed—as does the modern mind—from the known to the unknown. The cave man knew that when *he* struck an animal or another human down, it was because he *intended* to do so. There was a purpose, a person with destructive intentions, behind the act. Perhaps, then, there were similar but unseen persons, or spirits like persons, behind the mysterious blows which caused disease. This seemed highly probable to early man because of his whole outlook on the world around him.

Men had early conceived of souls or spirits which animated their own bodies but which could also exist outside thereof. For example, during dreams it seemed as if a man's soul left his sleeping body and moved about independently of it. In dreams he saw and talked with other men at a distance or even with those long dead. Ergo, men's souls must survive after death. These might well hover about their old homes and influence the living for good or ill.

Such explanations were applied to more than human behavior. Animals as well as men, and even many natural objects, moved about and seemed to have a life of their own. Perhaps these also were animated by inner spirits, even as were men. In a word, man projected his own consciousness into the world about him and pictured

8

spirits like his own in animals and birds, in woods and hills, and even in the empty air throughout. This outlook, strange as it seems at first glance, can also be understood by recalling vestiges of it which survive in modern thought. We still speak poetically of "ole man river" or of the "spirit of the hills," and we tell children about supernatural beings in every fairy tale.

Since he lived, as it were, in two worlds—the visible and the invisible—primitive man had to adjust his ways to the one as well as to the other. Spirits, like visible things, might do him good or harm. They might, for example, cause disease. Some of them were believed to be evil by nature and these demons were always making trouble. But in other cases, men might offend certain spirits and so bring trouble on themselves. If a man violated a tribal rule or taboo, ancestors or other spirits guarding over the tribe would punish him by illness.

Again, a man's enemy might seek to injure him by enlisting the aid of a demon. Rituals and incantations were formulated for this purpose. Spells were cast, for example, by sticking sharp objects into an image of the victim. Knowledge of such procedures was known as "black magic" and its practice survived into modern times. Eventually, it was combined with various religious doctrines in so-called witchcraft, and witchcraft cases occasionally come up in courts even at the present time.

Invisible agencies were believed to cause sickness in still other ways. Besides using spells at a distance, demons might force small stones or animals into their victims or a devil might himself invade a man's body. In that case the latter was said to be possessed (controlled) by the evil spirit, and this later became one explanation of the strange behavior of the insane. One still says of a difficult child, "I can't imagine what possesses him."

Illness, of course, was not the only injury inflicted on men by offended or evil spirits. The causes of most dangers that beset mankind were ascribed to invisible influences. Floods, storms, attacks by animals—all of these might have a magic origin. No wonder that early men lived in terror of the unseen. We can still sense such a feeling if we are caught in mysterious surroundings. Graveyards at midnight (where the dead hover), the howling of a distant dog on a lonely moor, the creaking door in a "haunted house"—all these may bring back something of this ancient fear.

Yet there might be means of protection. It was logical to seek magical defenses against magical dangers. Offended spirits could be placated by offerings or ceremonies and demons could be met by magic words or objects which would frighten them off—by barriers they did not dare to pass. These charms were tried and often no harm followed. Then, by the same reasoning that was applied to experience with drugs, it was concluded that safety was conferred by the particular charm employed. This might be an object supposed to ward off danger of any kind (amulet) ; or it could be one which—like a horseshoe or rabbit's foot today—brought good luck in general (talisman).

If one feared a demon or spell which brought illness in a particular body part, a charm representing that part might provide protection. Or if one dreaded the "evil eye" of an enemy—and a penetrating glance might seem a real menace—an amulet portraying this organ might counteract the threat. Hundreds of such objects have been found in the debris of prehistoric dwellings.

If charms failed, evil spirits might be appeased by special gifts. At times, too, solely physical ways of getting rid of demons were employed. It has been suggested that repulsive medicines were first given to disgust a possessing spirit and so drive him out. Patients were also prodded and rolled about, apparently in the same hope that this would expel the troublemaker. Massage is said to have originated in this sort of practice. The general idea survives in modern expressions, as in the none-too-elegant remark about "knocking the devil out of him."

Alongside the lore about evil influences there also grew up a belief in good spirits. A man helped his family or friends and it seemed likely that there were friendly beings who shared such benevolent intentions. Their aid was solicited and charms or offerings for this purpose were evolved. When enemies cast evil spells, counterspells could be formulated. Thus arose what became known as good or "white magic."

Both black and white magic could be at work at the same time, and the individual who was caught between them had to "watch his step" with the greatest care. Some African tribesmen are known to spend an hour or two each day in arranging charms or counter-charms, before they dare to go about their business. Our own fairy tales are reminiscent of this situation. In the story, "Snow White and the Seven Dwarfs," the Wicked Queen directs black magic against the heroine, who is in turn protected by the white variety. Suspense is provided by the awful uncertainty—right down to the last chapter or scene—as to which type of magic will prove the stronger.

Men thus oriented their lives in relation to two worlds, the visible and the invisible. And they adjusted themselves to the latter largely in terms of two kinds of magic. In so far as this adjustment concerned protection against illness, the resulting practices are known as "magic medicine." This did not replace the natural medicine of drugs and surgery, but was added to or combined with it.

The practice of modern primitives suggests that simple illnesses were either ignored or treated with natural drugs, while serious illness demanded a search for the cause and therefore for magical measures. But it may be that both types of treatment were, at times, used simultaneously. Such a combining of natural and occult elements is not so different, after all, from what is sometimes done today in our own society. The midwife, mentioned earlier, employs natural medical procedures at the same time that she sets amulets about and so provides the right supernatural setting.

The Medicine Man

Having explained something about early man's concept of illness and about the means he found for dealing with it, one may proceed to the question of how the sick actually were treated. Like the aged, the ill are always a problem. They cannot produce for themselves and may take the time of others. This could be very serious for a small group of savages who needed all their resources—the energies of all their members—if they were to survive. Yet we cannot assume that early man was always callous in his attitude toward sick fellows or that he simply got rid of them as so many burdens. The virtues of sympathy and mercy were displayed by some uncivilized peoples, and were not necessarily practiced more often as civilization advanced.

As a rule, savages in the early cultural stage of hunting and fishing extended some care to invalids and the infirm. They gave them a share of the food—which was common property of the tribe— and carried them along on migrations when possible. Such care undoubtedly involved what could be called the beginnings of nursing, although it was simply provided by the invalid's family or friends. Originally, this behavior also may have begun on the animal level; apes, for example, are known to show sympathy for one of their number who is ill. But in human behavior sympathy was expressed in service, which was incorporated in the customs of a given people.

Just who provided rudimentary nursing probably varied with the customs of each group or tribe. Civilized experience suggests that women are usually more considerate of the helpless than are men. It therefore may be held that women are better adapted biologically to care for invalids; but individual differences within either sex must also be taken into account. So, too, must the roles assigned to each sex by any given society. No clear pattern emerges here. Early men, in general, did not allocate the care of the sick to either men or women as such.

Some modern primitives not only looked after those who were ill but also accorded them special recognition. Certain North American Indian tribes, for example, regarded those who had recovered from acute illness with great respect. These individuals were thought to have been close to the spirit world and were believed to have acquired wisdom in consequence. If mentally ill, moreover, their strange behavior was viewed as a result of direct contacts with spirits, and they were therefore venerated as peculiarly inspired persons.

In contrast to such attitudes, other primitives were ruthless in their treatment of both the chronically ill and of the aged. This was apt to be true of more advanced pastoral or agricultural peoples, who held private property and were not inclined to share it readily with handicapped individuals. Such persons were abandoned or killed as useless burdens, or might be expected to commit suicide. Even such peoples, however, made efforts to care for those of the sick who apparently had a chance for recovery.

Actual procedure in such cases varied with the seriousness of the illness. Minor or commonplace conditions were, as noted, probably left to take care of themselves—much as we often do with the common cold. Or this may have been the sort of thing which was handled through the use of natural remedies, such as emetics or purgatives. Acute illness, on the other hand, called for special action. Something unusual and occult was clearly at work, and it was in such an emergency that the cause must be identified. Magic medicine then came into play.

Within a very primitive group, occult measures may have been taken by the victim himself or by his family. Or perhaps the elders of the group were called in consultation. They would question the afflicted person, inquiring how he might have offended the ancestors or other spirits by breaking some tribal rule or taboo. Or was he the victim of certain demons or of a spell cast by an enemy? In the first instance, offerings or prayers would be made by way of propitiation; in the second, counter-spells or incantations must be carried out to ward off the evil influence. These ceremonies were conducted by the sick man or by various onlookers; there was as yet no individual who specialized in such healing.

As magic lore accumulated, however, it became too complex for the knowledge and understanding of the ordinary tribesman. Certain individuals who were supposed to have special insight, or peculiar contacts with spirits, then devoted time to mastering this lore and to interpreting it for the benefit of their fellows. In order to qualify for this role, a man might have to go through some mystical experience, perhaps going into trances or spending weeks alone in communion with the spirit world. He thus became a dedicated person, set off from others and instructed by some older man who played the same part. Here was the beginning of specialization in the art of healing.

Any man who devoted himself to helping the sick doubtless became an authority on the folk medicine of the tribe. This included not only simple remedies (therapy) but also some knowledge from experience of where illnesses seemed to be located and what their outcome was likely to be (prognosis). It is not clear, however, that primitive healers had any notion of the existence of different diseases; they probably distinguished only between mild and acute conditions in general. The problem, in acute cases, was not to give the illness a name but to find a cure. And as noted, this required that the healer identify the magical cause in order to overcome it. Hence, although familiar with folk medicine, the healer was primarily concerned with occult lore and procedures.

North American Indians possessed healers of this type, and their ceremonies were observed by early settlers in the English colonies. Noting that such men played a role analogous to that of physicians,

13

the English called them "medicine men" and the name has stuck. As will be explained later, the European medical practice of the 1600's was none too effective, and some colonists were glad to secure remedies from the medicine men when their own seemed useless. Thus, during the early history of this country, a primitive type of healing actually competed at times with European practice.

Usually, however, it was the naturalistic elements in Indian medicine—the roots and herbs or other drugs—which appealed to the Europeans. The magic elements made less impression. Colonials were familiar with occult lore and often believed in their own version thereof, but they found Indian magic meaningless. Yet it was the magic which meant most to primitives—not only to the medicine men but to their patients as well. Strange as the spells and incantations seemed to Europeans, they were taken as seriously by the primitives as we today take the procedures of science.

The more dramatic or mysterious the medicine man was, the more awed were the observers. This must have tempted the healer to "put up a front"—to introduce mystery or hocus-pocus just to increase his hold on the others. All professional men, including modern doctors, are tempted in this direction. But one could just as well reverse this analysis and say that the medicine man—like the modern physician in some cases—only gave his people what they wanted. They expected him to put on an act. It is also to be remembered that the weird behavior of medicine men was intended to drive out spirits who, it was believed, would resist any milder measures.

Here is an account of a medicine man's actual procedures, taken from George Catlin's descriptions of Indians as late as the 1830's. He had witnessed a battle between the Blackfoot and Cree tribes, in which a chief of the former was seriously wounded. Referring to the Blackfoot medicine man, who was called to the dying chief, Catlin wrote as follows:

> . . . his body and head were entirely covered with the skin of
> a yellow bear, the head of which (his own head being inside
> of it) served as a mask; the huge claws of which also, were
> dangling on his wrists and ankles; in one hand he shook a
> frightful rattle, and in the other brandished his medicine
> spear or magic wand; to the rattling din and discord of all of
> which, he added the wild and startling jumps and yelps of the
> Indian, and the horrid and appalling grunts, and snarls, and

growls of the grizzly bear, in ejaculatory and gutteral incantations to the Good and Bad Spirits, in behalf of his patient;
who was rolling and groaning in the agonies of death, whilst
he was dancing around him, jumping over him, and pawing
him about, and rolling him in every direction. . . .

A spectacle of this sort would hardly do much for a modern
patient in the same situation. We would prescribe rest and quiet
rather than "pawing him about"—transfusions rather than terroriza-
tion. And, even in Catlin's case, the rough handling and general hulla-
baloo may well have hastened the death of the victim.

In less extreme cases, however, the medicine man may have been
of some service. Sick persons, then as now, liked to feel that everything
possible was being done for them; and no one could accuse the medicine man of neglecting his patient. The latter, having faith in the
incantations, began to hope for a cure. And this improvement in
morale, in turn, might sometimes turn the scales in favor of recovery.

The modern physician, of course, has much more to offer. Yet
even the wise, present-day doctor—like the ancient healer—is aware
of old truths and therefore seeks to inspire confidence in his patient.
It is a far cry from the dramatics of the medicine man to the bedside
manner of contemporary practice; but the psychologic basis of both
approaches is, in the long run, much the same.

Religious Healing

The account here given of primitive medicine has noted only its
naturalistic and occult elements; nothing has been said as yet of
religious healing. In so far as early men believed in good spirits who
were more powerful than ordinary demons and who ruled over all
things, we may say that their ideas took on a religious nature. And
if any of them believed in a supreme being or beings, they certainly
appealed to them for aid against illness as against other dangers. But
primitives probably did not make such distinctions between magic
and religion as we would today; both were parts of their general
relation to the unseen.

It seems likely, nevertheless, that early men were confronted by
truly religious questions. Mention has been made of their belief in
the survival of souls after death, which is indicated by various burial
practices. Prehistoric Peruvians, as well as the Egyptians, preserved

15

the bodies of the dead in apparent belief that these would be needed by souls in the hereafter. And many early peoples enclosed in their burial mounds various articles to serve their owners in the last, great voyage into the unknown. Even cave men faced the mystery of death, which must have raised eternal problems in untutored minds.

Why was death inevitable and what became of souls thereafter? Could individuals do ought to postpone this tragedy or to assure themselves of immortality when it came? There were also questions about the group or tribe; what of its survival or destruction? The future, in all such matters, was uncertain and yet men wished desperately to know. Perhaps certain individuals might have peculiar insight into these mysteries—"second sight" or powers of divination. In due time, men who claimed to know the answers—who could speak on human destiny and what the future would bring—became a group apart even as had the medicine men. On the occult level they were known as wizards or soothsayers; but in a truly religious setting they became the priests and prophets who appeared in all early civilizations.

As implied above, it is not clear that primitives made distinctions between priests and medicine men. The same individual may have served in both capacities as the tribal authority on all the uncertainties of life. Or religious rites may have been practiced by the entire tribal troup, without designated leadership. But the earliest records, notably those of Egypt, reveal societies which possessed both priests and physicians. Religious and medical activities were thus differentiated, among some peoples, at a quite early period.

The distinction, nevertheless, was still not as sharp as it would become eventually. Both priests and physicians dealt with problems of life and death and both were authorities on traditional lore. For this reason, either might encroach on the other's field as we now define it. Priests might make healing more and more a religious matter, while physicians might attempt explanations of eternal mysteries. Down into recent centuries, priests accused doctors of undermining religion; while physicians were critical of those who promised religious healing.

This does not mean that physicians and priests were always in conflict. They usually participated harmoniously—or at least with little friction—in the affairs of a common culture. Their relationships must be noted, nevertheless, because there was a tendency in some ancient societies for priests to take over many medical functions. As religion became a complicated system, with great temples and elaborate ceremonies, religious healing frequently impressed men more than did ordinary, lay medical services.

In relation to really primitive medicine, however, all this was a late development that came only with the establishment of complex social institutions. Religion, magic, and naturalistic medicine were all present by that time—in combination or in isolation as the case might be. This is the stage that will be encountered when the first great civilizations are considered in ensuing chapters. The cultures of Egypt, India, Mesopotamia, China—and finally of Greece and Rome—all exhibited these several elements in their medical traditions.

Since each of these traditions had evolved slowly from prehistoric beginnings, no one of them can be understood save against the background of primitive medicine as just described. Lacking this, it would not be possible to explain the eventual appearance of true medical science. Such science had its remote origins in primitive observations, was then given distinct form within the civilizations noted, and would finally—at long last—come to dominate medical thought as a whole.

Chapter II

Ancient Civilizations:

First Appearance of a Nursing Personnel

The early civilizations on which that of the modern western world is based, were those of the eastern Mediterranean area. In Egypt, Syria, Mesopotamia, and even further east in India, oriental peoples developed cultures of a high order long before anything similar appeared in most parts of the world.[1] Some of their buildings, such as the Egyptian pyramids, still stand today although more than four thousand years old. By comparison, a so-called "oldest house" in the United States, which is at most three to four hundred years old, seems practically a modern building. This does not mean, however, that the United States is altogether a new nation. Much of our own culture goes back to and is therefore as old as the ancient traditions of the Near East.

The arts and learning of primitive men slowly evolved through what is termed the stone age, when all tools were made of stone or bone, into a so-called iron age when the use of several metals was added. With these advantages others were acquired, notably the domestication of plants and animals. It was found that certain wild grasses, such as wheat or rye, could be cultivated as cereals, and that certain animals such as sheep could be used for food and clothing.

[1] Early civilizations also appeared in China and Japan, but these long had no direct contacts with the Western World and exerted little influence upon it. Even more isolated were the ancient cultures which American Indians developed in Mexico and Peru.

Others, such as horses, could be employed as draught animals. (So impressive was their strength compared to that of men, that we still refer to the work of machines in terms of "horsepower.") These improvements made it possible to give up a life of nomadic hunting and to settle down as herdsmen and farmers. And this way of living, with materials for food and clothing always at hand, provided leisure to develop the arts and crafts. What is now called "progress" began to pick up a little momentum.

This was particularly true in regions where the soil and climate encouraged farming and where easily tamed animals were available. Hence it was no accident that the first great civilizations developed in the warm, rich river valleys of the Nile, the Euphrates, and the Indus; while in cold regions like northern Europe man continued to gain a precarious living as a hunter and his culture remained at a barbaric level.

Egyptian Civilization

One of the first civilizations to emerge clearly from barbarism was that of Egypt. It is well recalled today, because it left behind such impressive and enduring monuments to its former grandeur. The pyramids, tombs and temples along the Nile are still among the wonders of the contemporary world. Formal records, carved in solid stone or written in inks on paper scrolls called papyri, tell more about this ancient culture than do the buildings themselves. For two thousand years or more it was impossible to read these writings, since the very language and signs were long forgotten. Many a traveler stood in awe to observe

Among the ruined temples there,
Stupendous columns, and wild images
Of more than man, where marble daemons watch
The Zodiac's brazen mystery, and dead men
Hang their mute thoughts on the mute walls around.

Early in the last century, however, clues were found in the famous Rosetta Stone which enabled scholars to decipher the inscriptions. This was a stone on which the same record was inscribed in both the Greek and Egyptian languages; and since the former was well known, it was possible by comparison to figure out the meaning of the latter. Thus a key was discovered which unlocked all Egyptian writings. Similiar keys were later discovered for other early inscriptions like the Babylonian, but a number of important ancient languages—for example, Cretan, and the American Mayan and Aztec carvings—remain largely unreadable to this day.

Surviving Egyptian records relate to periods as remote as 3,000 B.C. As might be expected, they reveal an already complex civilization, itself the product of still earlier centuries. There was a thriving economic life, based on agriculture and trade; all sorts of practical arts were developed; family and other social relationships were maintained along lines laid down by accepted moral codes; and the whole society was held together by an absolute monarchy under the "pharaoh" or king. Five thousand years ago these people doubtless considered themselves the last word in culture, as they looked back on their already ancient past. Such vanity may be pardoned in a people who had raised their monuments nearly five hundred feet into the sky. Some appreciation of their interests, skills, and ways of living may be secured today by looking at collections of Egyptian materials, such as those in the exhibits of the Metropolitan Museum in New York City.

What was the medical aspect of this ancient civilization? Or, to be more specific, from what diseases did the Egyptians suffer, what groups or professions cared for the sick, and what was the nature of their medical practice? Was this a matter of folk wisdom, or magic, or priestly lore, or of science as we now understand the term? Such questions may be applied to any particular culture, in order to "break down" or analyze the whole medical phase of its activities.

It is impossible to give simple answers for a history which extends, as does that of the Nile valley, over several millennia. In the earlier periods, Egyptian medicine seems to have included both folk practice and the usual magic, but it later exhibited some interest in natural science. All of these elements were also combined, at times, with the religious beliefs and rituals which played a central role in Egyptian life.

The religion of the Nile valley cultivated many gods, and eventually the power to both cause and cure disease was ascribed to these deities. This brought some order out of the old confusion about innumerable demons, which was associated with earlier, magic medicine. For now there were but a few beings who must be propitiated.

21

Moreover, as priests built temples to these gods, they developed traditions of worship and well-established ways of requesting divine aid for the sick. These rituals preserved something of folk remedies or magical procedures, but they were all united in a single religious cult. The special god of healing was Imhotep, who was probably originally a real person—perhaps a king or priest unusually skilled in medicine. People flocked to his temples for healing and so these became sanctuaries for the sick. One might almost view them as the first sanatoriums.

It happened that Egyptian religion was especially concerned with the question of life after death. More than any other ancient race, these people hoped for personal survival beyond the grave. The pyramid was their symbol for immortality, and it survives to this day not only in the famous Washington Monument but also at the top of the other obelisks that dot our many cemeteries. To make doubly sure of personal survival, bodies were skillfully embalmed so that souls could remain therein or return to them when the after-life began. These mummies have been preserved to our own time and provide a unique opportunity to study the conditions which caused sickness or death so long ago. Numerous autopsies have been performed on mummies which were several thousand years old, almost as they might be performed upon ordinary subjects today. The results have been enlightening. Lesions showing the existence of such diseases as tuberculosis and arteriosclerosis have been found in bodies of 1,000 B.C., along with indication of parasitic infections. Many of the ills now common plagued these ancient folk, though there is no proof that all contemporary diseases were present.

A picture of Egyptian medicine at its best is preserved in several famous medical papyri. There are three elements in these manuscripts, religion and magic on the one hand and matter-of-fact accounts of sickness and treatment on the other. This combination appears strange to us, but it probably seemed natural enough to the original authors. Or it may be that the two elements were written at different periods, or by different professions—as by priests in some cases and by lay physicians in others. The latter seemed to have practiced even when temple cults were active, so that two professions—doctors and priests—dealt with the sick at the same time although in different ways. But there is no mention of nurses or of other additional medical personnel.

Those portions of the papyri which describe illness in purely natural terms may be said to represent the beginnings of scientific medicine. In the first place, this was obviously different from magic with its supernaturalism. In the second place, it differed also from folk medicine. The latter may be practical enough and in some respects quite sound, but tends to become an unreasoning tradition in which it is impossible to separate sense from nonsense. Folk medicine was just a collection of supposed cures piled on top of each other with no theory or system whatever. Egyptian scientific medicine possessed, in contrast, some ideas about anatomy and physiology, about disease causation, and about prevention and cures. These theories bound the whole together. We would say that there was some sense to it. In a word, science must be rational and systematic as well as naturalistic in its procedures.

Whether medical science grew originally out of folk medicine or rather out of priestly lore, is difficult to determine. Perhaps it had roots in both fields. It seems likely, however, that lay doctors developed the beginnings of science directly out of folk practice; whereas priestly medicine went off in a different direction that was to constitute the tradition of religious healing. Both this sort of healing and real science tended to become separated from folk medicine, in part because the latter was maintained by humble, illiterate persons and lost prestige in consequence. The subsequent isolation of folk practice from that of physicians was probably unfortunate for both forms. Thus folk medicine became degraded and despised by the learned, while the doctors overlooked practical remedies which the plain people could have contributed. This point will be raised again in connection with modern medicine; but in the meantime, the actual beginnings of scientific medicine along the Nile may be briefly considered.

The papyri show that Egyptians had some elementary knowledge of gross anatomy, as of the heart and great vessels. Such knowledge was probably acquired from animal dissections rather than from preparing mummies, for in the latter process the human organs were not handled with any care. Physicians had their theories about physiology, ascribing much importance to the heart and blood, and also to the brain (which is remarkable in view of its lack of sound or motion). Their ideas about disease causation emphasized the danger of parasitic infections, which seems natural enough in a tropical region. Of pathologic processes they knew little, save of such obvious changes as "hardening in the limbs" (arthritis deformans).

Yet the Egyptian physicians did give names to various ills, which suggests that they thought they could distinguish between diverse clinical pictures in terms of body parts and symptoms. This awareness of different diseases would prove important in later medicine and the first signs of it in Egypt are therefore significant. The Greek historian, Herodotus, even declared that Egyptian physicians specialized in treating particular diseases—each body part having doctors who dealt with it alone. If so, this is the earliest appearance of specialization, and represents a professional arrangement to which we have returned in some measure within the last half century.

In seeking to diagnose special diseases, Egyptian practitioners employed general observation and such simple procedures as palpation. Because of their interest in the heart, the pulse was also noted. Long sections in the papyri give directions to the doctor, and these involve diagnosis as well as anatomy, therapy, and prognosis. The following is a selection from the Ebers Papyrus which illustrates the doctor's mode of procedure and the sort of learning he employed:[2]

CLINICAL EVIDENCE	If you examine a person who suffers from pains in the stomach, and is sick in the breast and the stomach, and it appears that
DIAGNOSIS	it is the disease *UAT,* you will say: "Death has entered into thy mouth" . . . You will
PHARMACY THERAPEUTICS	prepare a remedy composed of the following plants. . . . You will have them cooked in beer. . . . You will give it to the sick person
PROGNOSIS	to drink, then you will put your hands on the sick person and his arm will be extended without pain, and then you will say: "The disease has gone out from the intestine . . . it is not necessary to repeat the medicine."

These directions may seem a bit vague to us now, but note their complete freedom from magic and superstition. Observe also the forbearance in not repeating the medicine—a restraint which was rare in the practice of some later periods.

A high level of ancient practice was reached in the Egyptian surgery of about 2,500 B.C. This is revealed in the Edwin Smith Papyrus, translated by the American orientalist James Breasted in 1930.

2 Quoted in Arturo Castiglioni, *History of Medicine,* edited and translated by E. B. Krumbhaar, New York, Alfred A. Knopf, Inc., 1947, p. 53.

Here was a text book on surgery arranged according to the general parts of the body, of which only the section relating to the upper parts survives. The clinical observations are fairly accurate and the surgical directions so adequate that it is difficult to realize that it was written five thousand years ago. The care of fractures with splints, the reduction of dislocations, and the general treatment of wounds are all covered in minute detail. Much attention is given to methods of bandaging. There is some knowledge of the suturing of wounds and even mention of the possibilities of plastic surgery. Minor operations, such as the removal of obvious tumors, are described. Although there is no reference to major operations, it should be remembered that the surgery of all periods prior to the last century was largely limited to superficial procedures.

Notable in this Papyrus also is the absence of magic which is mentioned but once in the entire work. So, too, is its objective spirit. Frequently it is observed, in the prognosis attached to each case: "Nothing can be done," or "The patient will die." Magicians would rarely make such an admission; quacks, never. Here was the spirit of true science.

Equally free from superstition were Egyptian ideas concerning personal hygiene. Indeed, both surgery and hygiene long exhibited more common sense than did internal medicine, perhaps because the latter necessarily related to mysterious matters. Anyone could see that a splint was effective, or realize that cleanliness was pleasant and apparently a protection from disease; whereas what happened when a drug went into the body was a pretty obscure affair.

Living in a tropical region, the Egyptians developed strict rules about such matters as cleanliness, exercise, food, drink, and sex relations. These rules were stated in terms of religious authority but their hygienic values were obvious. Priests, for example, could drink only boiled or filtered water—a precaution which, if observed in our own times, would have saved thousands of lives as late as 1900. Special attention was given to the hygiene of infants who, after weaning, were given cow's milk and fresh vegetables. This also seems up to date. It is one of the ironies of history that certain "modern" ideas or practices appeared so long ago, only to be lost or deliberately discarded until revived in recent days.

As a matter of fact, Egyptian medical history itself illustrates this tendency for it is not a story of continual progress. There is said to have been more magic and less science in the medicine of 500 B.C. than there had been in that of 2,500 B.C. Certain kinds of knowledge continued to accumulate but this was not an unmixed blessing. The pharmacopoeia, for example, became so complicated that it must have been confusing and largely useless. More than seven hundred drugs were eventually listed and this was altogether too many for an ancient people to handle intelligently. Just why this decadence occurred is not easily explained, and in any case an attempt to do so would require a study of the whole history of the country that is beyond the present purpose. Not until Greek culture flourished in Alexandria a few centuries before Christ, would Egypt again become a center of medical progress.

Developments in Mesopotamia

Side by side with Egyptian civilization had developed that of ancient Mesopotamia. This was a Greek word meaning "between the rivers"; that is, the land between the Tigris and the Euphrates in the region now known as Iraq. Here, just as along the Nile, a well-watered soil and warm climate encouraged the early appearance of advanced civilizations. One after another rose and fell, as successive peoples came in from the surrounding deserts and conquered their predecessors in the fertile valleys. Sumerians, Assyrians, Babylonians, and Persians followed one another as the dominant people, in that chronological order. Conquerors took over the earlier civilizations, however, so that there was an accumulation of culture from the ancient Sumerian period about 3,000 B.C. down to the flowering of Persian life more than two thousand years later.

This progress frequently followed the same lines as those already noted in Egypt. There was the usual development of agriculture and trade, of practical arts, and of a system of written inscriptions. There were also, of course, certain differences. Mesopotamians built in soft clay or bricks instead of in stone. Hence nothing remains today of their ancient cities except mounds of debris, whereas Egyptian monuments still stand against the desert sky. Even the step-back skyscraper temples of Babylon—there is a description of one in the Biblical account of the Tower of Babel—have long since crumbled to dust. Fortunately, their writings were made on hardened clay tablets many of which are preserved in American museums. Until the last century no one could read these records; but, as in the case of Egyptian writing, clues were then found which made it possible to interpret the secrets hitherto locked up in wedge-shaped (cuneiform) inscriptions.

From these one can learn much of Assyrian and Babylonian religion, business and, most important here, of their medical practices. As in Egypt, Mesopotamian records reveal an early folk medicine which became overlaid with magic and was partly absorbed in priestly cults. Marduk and other gods held power over health and disease. Various occult practices, such as the art of divination, were cultivated. That art was not strictly medical but it might involve prognostication in illness as well as prophecy of other future events. But since it was supposed that the future could be read in animal organs, divination led to—or at least displayed—some anatomical information. Babylonian clay models of the liver, used for this purpose, are more accurate representations than those made three thousand years later during the Middle Ages. There is an account in the Bible of a Babylonian king who, in order to reach a major decision, "looked in the liver" to see what lay before him (Ezekiel, XXI, 21).

A more elaborate attempt to foresee the future appeared in astrology. The origins of this pseudo-science, which has come down to us from Babylon and which some Americans still take seriously, are obscure enough. Man must always have stood in awe of heavenly bodies set in the vast reaches of the sky. Everyone could see that life itself depended in some way upon the sun. Only less impressive was

> That orbèd maiden with white fire laden,
> Whom mortals call the moon.

Poets have long loved to personify her as Luna and in ancient days men really believed her to be a goddess—perhaps the consort of the sun-god. Both played a large role in ancient religions and we continue to name days of the week after them. Together they were associated with the alternation of day and night which so affected man's activities, and they also seemed to affect him in more subtle ways. Who has not felt the spell of the full moon? One heard of moon-struck lovers and of lunatics; that is, of those driven mad by Luna's rays.

The regular progress of the moon's phases, moreover, seemed to parallel the periodicity of physiological phenomena or of certain diseases like the periodic fevers. Perhaps the one caused the other; that is, the moon might actually exert some control over human affairs. Here was a possible clue to the problem which had always puzzled man—whence came the mysterious influences that controlled his body and even his luck or destiny? Not only the moon but the other bodies that moved across the sky might hold the answer. Certainly the stars were more real and impressive than petty demons, and their majestic regularity suggested vast and mysterious powers. Moreover, if the stars controlled men's lives, a study of them might yield their secrets and thus reveal the future. With this thought in mind, Babylonian priests became true stargazers and learned much about the sun, moon, and planets that would eventually become the basis of scientific astronomy. They were excellent mathematicians, a trait which they developed in the course of such studies, and they invented that system of measuring in units of sixty which is still employed in circular measurements—as in seconds, minutes, and hours on the face of a watch.

With the aid of mathematics, the priests noted the position of the "fixed stars" and the motions of the planets and the moon, and came to see in all these matters so many signs of their influence on men. As their lore accumulated, they began to "cast horoscopes" in terms of an individual's birth, for the position of the planets at this time was supposed to cast a spell over a man thereafter. To this day, we say that a person can "thank his lucky star" for some fortunate occurrence; and if something turns out badly, it is called "an ill-starred event."

It followed from all this that no important decision could be made without first consulting the stars to see if the signs were propitious. The king would not declare war, or the farmer begin his spring plowing, until he had found whether the stars were in a lucky position. To do the opposite was to fly in the face of ill omens. For the same reason men would not take remedies or employ other medical procedures unless the moon was in the right phase or the planets in proper conjunction. In this way medicine became all mixed up with astrology on the plains of Babylon some four thousand years ago, and it never became permanently disentangled therefrom until the last two centuries. As late as the time of the American colonies, physicians wrote books with such titles as "The Necessity of Astrology for Medicine." It would not be difficult, even today, to find folk who time the taking of medicines by the phases of the moon.

Such practices, which were in effect a special form of magic medicine, were in the hands of astrologer-priests. Here was a combination of magic, religion, and science all in the one cult and handled by one profession. Despite this, however, the clay tablets of Mesopotamia also show the survival of lay physicians. These men, as might be expected, were inclined to follow the empirical or trial-and-error practice which had originated in folk medicine. If their coexistence with astrological cults seems surprising, only remember again that various kinds of medicine, of magic, and of religious healing are still practiced side by side in contemporary society.

The lay physicians and surgeons of Babylon had their drugs and superficial surgery, supplemented no doubt by magical hocus-pocus for good measure. They had to be careful about their practice since they were held accountable for the consequences. Babylonian legal codes were more advanced than those of any ancient culture and regulated the responsibilities of every group. Particularly severe was the social control of surgeons. The famous Code of Hammurabi—inscribed about 1900 B.C. on a single stone shaft—provides that surgeons making successful incisions should be paid in silver, but should have their hands cut off if they caused the death of their patients! This was the "eye for an eye and a tooth for a tooth" morality which is also reported in the Bible. One presumes that there was little unnecessary surgery under these circumstances.

There was nothing notable in the internal medicine of the lay physicians but their clinical observations reveal a fairly accurate portrayal of symptoms. The diseases involved can sometimes be recognized, as in the following statement which suggests bronchitis or some other pulmonary condition:[3]

> The sick one coughs frequently, his sputum is thick, his respirations give a sound like a flute.

Brief as this is, it affords a better clinical picture than the mere statement, quoted above from an Egyptian papyrus, that the patient "suffers from pains in the stomach" and so on. One might view these accounts as early case records. These may have been of no help in themselves to patients, but they reveal a desire to describe disease phenomena as objectively as possible.

[3] Castiglioni, *History of Medicine*, 39.

Herodotus declared that Babylonians put their sick out in public places, so that all who passed could examine them and suggest diagnoses and cures. Here was folk medicine on a wholesale scale. Whether such public clinical discussions were actually held is a question, but the story at least suggests that emphasis was placed upon repeated examinations of patients. For all their magic, the Babylonians were evidently an observant people. This appeared in their medicine as well as in astronomy. Consumed with curiosity concerning the world about them, they left some of the best ancient accounts of "the heavens above, the earth beneath, and the waters under the earth."

Early Jewish Contributions

By the later Babylonian period, after 1500 B.C., contacts between the various cultures of the Near East became closer and more continuous. Something was known of Egyptian medicine in Mesopotamia and vice versa. A series of civilizations developed in the so-called "Fertile Crescent"; that is, in the area that stretched from the Isthmus of Suez (where contact was made with Egypt) up through Palestine and Syria, east through the region of Damascus, and then down the Euphrates Valley. On the western side of this crescent opposite Mesopotamia, and separated from the latter by the deserts east of Jerusalem, appeared the civilizations of the Phoenicians and of the Jews. North of these was the Aramaic culture of Syria, which centered in Damascus. Most of these peoples, like the Babylonians, spoke so-called Semitic languages. Hebrew was one, but by the time of Christ the Jews had given up their own language and were speaking Aramaic.

Their position between Egypt on the one hand, and Syria and Mesopotamia on the other, made the ancient Jewish peoples a go-between for these two cultural areas and contributed much to their own civilization. The Jews were the first to develop the art of writing historical narratives and these early histories are preserved in the Old Testament. In Genesis, Exodus and other books, we are told how Abraham (Israel) first came into Palestine, how his descendants (the "Children of Israel") were made captives in Egypt, how they escaped therefrom into Palestine, how they were then conquered and taken into exile "by the waters of Babylon," and how the Persians finally restored them to Jerusalem. In the course of these adventures they absorbed much of the culture of both Egypt and Babylon, and the Bible is full of accounts of those two civilizations.

The early Jews made little contribution to either internal medicine or surgery. The Bible reveals, for example, no surgery comparable to that of the more ancient Egyptians. On the other hand, Jewish religion was associated with a notable development of personal and public hygiene. This, in turn, was to have an influence on the later Christians through their use of the Jewish scriptures.

The religious leaders of Palestine were among the first to renounce a belief in many gods, in order to worship what they believed was the one true God. "Thou shalt have no other Gods but Me," declares the First Commandment. This monotheistic conception had been formed in Egypt at an earlier period but had exerted only temporary influence there. Now the Jews permanently established the belief that all power over life and death was in the hands of Jehovah. Hence they repudiated the magic and astrology which were practiced all around them. Their priests taught that the preservation of health, as well as all other values in life, was to be found simply in "keeping pure before the Lord." This did not call for any particular medical practices, but rather for a way of living directed by the priests and incorporated in the Mosaic Law.

This code enforced rules which, though expressed in religious terms, had definite hygienic significance. Certain animal foods such as pork were declared unclean and therefore were forbidden. Exact directions for handling those meats permitted for food were provided, and these have been observed ever since in the kosher regulations of orthodox Jews. Since pork is dangerous as a source of parasitic infections, the value of its prohibition is obvious.

The Mosaic Law also provided regulations for the general welfare, as can be seen in directions for the sanitary police of military camps. But the most interesting phase of Jewish hygiene was the belief that certain diseases were "unclean before the Lord" and that these might be acquired by contact with unclean peoples. Thus their soldiers were warned against the women of conquered peoples, lest they be defiled by venereal infections. This idea of infection by contact (contagion) seems obvious enough now but the Jews were unusual among ancient peoples in emphasizing it. Note that it was really a naturalistic concept. While others might give magical explanations of how demons or gods caused epidemic diseases, the Israelites concluded that these spread from one individual to the next. Hence the way to prevent them was to avoid contacts.

The most elaborate formulation of contagion doctrine related to the disease of leprosy. This was not the same infection as the one now called by that name, but was certainly a lingering and finally fatal condition. It exhibited revolting superficial lesions and was widespread throughout the ancient East. Detailed directions were provided, in the Bible, as to how contact with lepers and even with their clothing was to be avoided. Lepers were required to live apart and to cry "unclean," so as to identify themselves when approached by others. (Anyone who has read Lew Wallace's novel "Ben Hur" will recall the vivid portrayal of lepers in this role.) Thus the Jews not only pioneered in establishing the concept of contagion but also in those measures of notification and isolation which were based upon it. This approach to public health control, however, made little impression on other ancient races, and it remained for European Christians to revive it during the Middle Ages.

The Persian Empire

The Persians, who finally conquered Babylonia and enabled the Jews to return to Jerusalem, came into Mesopotamia from the grazing lands to the East. Iran, the present name of their country, is a form of the word "Aryan" and indicates that they spoke a so-called Indo-European or Aryan language. As far as one can tell from this language, the Persians were related to European peoples rather than to the old Semitic stocks of the Near East. The Persians, by about 500 B.C., conquered all of the Fertile Crescent and Egypt as well, so that they founded the most extensive Empire which had appeared in the Near East.

They absorbed much of the culture of the several conquered lands, among other things the medicine and surgery of Egypt. The Emperor Darius, for example, restored an old school for training priest-physicians in the Nile Delta. He repaired the buildings and provided surgical instruments and even students because (as his inscription states) "he knew the value of this art in order to save the life of everyone having sickness." This statement about the power of doctors to save everyone seems a bit optimistic, but at least it illustrates the degree of confidence which existed in Egyptian medicine. This is said to have been the first instance, by the way, in which a medical center was established as a royal or government foundation. But there is little of special interest in the medical history of the Persian Empire.

Medical Achievements in Ancient India

More significant is the story of another great branch of the Aryan peoples, which migrated into the Indus Valley of northwestern India. There they developed an advanced culture which was in contact with that of Persia to the West and indirectly with that of China to the East. Like the Persians, these people spoke an Indo-European language (Sanscrit), and their sacred books (the *Vedas*) are among the oldest writings now in existence. These are usually dated at about 1600 B.C., and it is not surprising to find in them the usual belief in magic medicine and in the divine control of health and disease. There were also special medical writings prepared in Sanscrit during the next millennium but these have been lost. Hence we have little direct knowledge of Indian medicine during the very periods when Babylonian and Jewish cultures were at their height.

Eventually a number of compendiums (*samhitas*) of the earlier medical works were prepared and these preserve something of the earlier medical writings. Of these collections, the most important were a surgical work called *Sushruta Samhita* and a medical manuscript entitled *Charaka Samhita*. No one knows their exact dates, which have been variously set all the way from about 500 B.C. to 400 A.D. They reveal suddenly, as it were, a highly developed medicine and surgery. This had no doubt developed slowly during the thousand years after the writing of the *Vedas,* partly as a result of contacts with the cultures of the Near East. If the later dates are accepted, Sanscrit medicine may also have owed something to Greek science, since Alexander the Great reached India in his conquests of 325 B.C. and added the Indus Valley to his great Empire. Conversely, Indian medicine may have influenced that of Greece; and some recent Hindu writers have claimed that European medicine was originally based largely upon that of India.

Lay physicians, as described in the *Sushruta Samhita,* were drawn from the upper castes—that is, from descendants of the Aryan conquerors who ruled over the original, dark-skinned natives. Great emphasis was placed upon the personal purity and devotion of the practitioner. The following description of a doctor seems a bit quaint but illustrates the ideal:[4]

[4] K. K. L. Bhishagratna, editor, *Sushruta Samhita,* I, Calcutta, 1907, p. 74.

> He should be cleanly in his habits and well shaved, and should not allow his nails to grow. He should wear white garments, put on a pair of shoes, carry a stick and an umbrella in his hands, and walk about with a mild and benignant look as a friend of all created beings. . . . A physician should adjure the company of women, nor should he speak in private to them or joke with them.

Like most ancient physicians, these dignified gentlemen had only crude ideas about anatomy and somewhat fanciful notions of physiology. The blood vessels, for example, were supposed to carry air and the nerves were said to start from the umbilicus. Indian medicine displayed some interesting ideas about pathology, however, notably the belief that disease might be due to impurities in the body fluids or humors. This humoral pathology was emphasized, subsequently, by Greek physicians and so became a basic concept of all later European medicine. Hindu practice employed bloodletting in order to get rid of the impure fluids and also called to its assistance the usually complicated pharmacopoeia.

The hygiene and surgery of the Hindus were more empirical and probably more successful than their internal medicine. Like other tropical folk, they laid down careful rules for cleanliness and diet in terms of religious laws. Going further than the Jewish prohibition of certain meats, they eventually encouraged complete vegetarianism. Their surgery was the most skillful of any ancient culture, and involved operations unknown to the later Greeks and Romans, for example, tonsillectomies. They not only performed amputations but excised tumors, repaired hernias, and couched for cataract. All sorts of surgical instruments were invented and great care was taken in methods of washing and bandaging wounds. In short, they developed minor surgery to about as high a level as was possible as long as anatomical knowledge was limited and effective anesthetics and antiseptics were unknown. Even here they made an empirical beginning, for dressings were made as cleanly as possible, bedding was sterilized, and wines were used to produce some degree of insensibility.

Another significant achievement of Indian medicine was its provision for public services. Some sort of vital statistics were collected, dangerous diseases were reported, and—most notable of all—hospitals were established. These were the first, as far as is known, in world history. Nothing like them appeared in Europe until the Middle Ages.

It was probably no accident that the country possessing the most advanced surgery of the ancient world was also the first to provide hospitals. Surgeons long needed institutional facilities more than did general practitioners, and one can well imagine that it was the Hindu surgeons who first called for the hospitalization of their patients. Just how common this practice was, or how many hospitals existed, is not certain. One difficulty is that the Sanscrit word which has been translated as meaning hospital can also be interpreted as "pharmacy" or "dispensary"—a less ambitious connotation. Yet there is no question that hospitals of some kind were built. These were constructed at times by government order, staffed by government-paid physicians, and supplied with government stores. Thus early did state medicine become a reality.

Thus early, too, appeared the first special nursing group known to history. It was, presumably, the existence of hospitals that made this personnel necessary. As long as the sick remained at home, their care naturally fell to their families. But as soon as they were removed to an institution, the services of some attendants in addition to physicians were obviously called for. Consideration then had to be given immediately to two problems which have ever since been basic in all nursing programs: (1) how to secure nurses who would give devoted service, and (2) how to train them in carrying out this service in an efficient manner. The first was a matter of moral or religious ideals, the latter a scientific objective. These considerations, in turn, involved many questions concerning the relation of nurses to patients on the one hand and to physicians on the other.

It was clear that neither the moral nor the scientific ideal, cultivated alone, would be adequate. The most devoted attendant who was at the same time totally ignorant, would never make an effective nurse. On the other hand, the most skilled attendant who felt no sympathy for the patients and viewed the work merely as a source of income, would never provide the best service. Indian medicine approached these problems in the following manner, as stated in the *Charaka Samhita:*[5]

> In the first place a mansion must be constructed . . . spacious and roomy . . . After this should be secured a body of attendants of good behaviour, distinguished for purity or cleanliness

[5] *Ibid.*, section XV, 168 f.

35

of habits, attached to the person for whose service they are engaged, possessed of cleverness and skill, endued with kindness, skilled in every kind of service that a patient may require . . . clever in bathing or washing a patient . . . well skilled in making or cleaning beds . . . and skillful in waiting upon one that is ailing, and never unwilling to do any act that they be commanded to do.

In the *Sushruta Samhita,* the whole matter is summed up as follows:

The physician, the patient, the medicine, and the attendants are the four essential factors of a course of medical treatment.

Sushruta then describes the ideal character of each of these elements in turn. The physician, as noted, was to be well trained and of great purity. Medicine was collected under astrological controls. Drugs should be helpful, but at the same time pleasant and harmless even in an overdose. The patient ought to have religious faith and obey his doctor. It is also interesting to observe that the ideal patient "should have a curable type of disease"—something no doubt helpful to professional reputations. Or perhaps this simply meant that the hospitals did not take incurables. The description of the nurse repeats in substance what has been quoted above.

One can recognize here an elementary description of both the techniques and ideals of a nursing group. It is not clear whether the attendants were thought of as glorified servants or whether they were viewed as professional personnel. In all probability there was a mixture of both attitudes—a confusion that persisted through many later periods. But Indian hospitals and medical services at least anticipated in some ways our modern institutions and points of view. The chief exception to this is the fact that these first nurses were always men. The generally inferior position of women in Oriental societies may explain the discrimination. Whether this implies that only men were admitted to the hospitals is not clear.

In view of the lack of hospitals and of nursing services in the ancient Near East, it is surprising that contemporary India came so close to our modern practice and ideals. It also seems unfortunate that Indian achievements in this field were not taken over into the later civilization of Greece and Rome, on which that of medieval and modern Europe was in turn to be constructed.

Chapter III

Greek Culture:

Anticipations of Modern Medicine

Thousands of Americans visit Greece and Italy and see in those countries the ruins of the classical age. Though tired of sightseeing, they rarely forget their first view of the Parthenon or of the Colosseum. To climb in the latter building the same stairs that Roman crowds once mounted, and to gaze down across the same sweeping amphitheater, is a breath-taking experience in more senses than one. An imaginative traveler can picture this scene as it once was, with fifty thousand excited people cheering on beasts or gladiators in the arena below. More colorful and more cruel than any modern sports, these spectacles would make present games pale by comparison. Those who have read such a novel as *Quo Vadis,* or descriptions of "blood and sand" in Spanish bull-rings—survivals of Roman arenas—will recall the dramatic setting.

But the tourist actually sees only stone arches and usually focuses attention on the building itself. It is much like our own stadiums, for the simple reason that the latter are copied from it. And upon its walls, or on those of buildings nearby, appear inscriptions in the same letters and using partially similar words to those now employed in English. All this recalls the fact that our alphabet as well as much of our language was borrowed centuries ago from the same people who once crowded the Colosseum for a "Roman holiday." This structure, then, is the handiwork of men who had much in common with us. It is not, like some strange temple in Egypt or Babylon, the relic of a civilization so remote that we can hardly comprehend it.

The more a traveler examines Greek or Roman ruins the more he will realize their similarity to many present buildings. The massive arches of the Baths of Caracalla, for example, provided an approximate model for the Pennsylvania Railroad Station in New York City. Plans were not the only things secured from the baths of ancient Rome. During medieval days, men simply demolished magnificent walls to find building stone for their own dwellings. Such vandalism was symbolic of the whole relation of Greco-Roman civilization to our own. Our medieval ancestors first destroyed a large part of the classical heritage and then rebuilt civilization from the portions that survived.

In other words, when we consider "the glory that was Greece and the grandeur that was Rome" we are approaching our own times. Some historians date the advent of "modern history" with the story of these classical peoples; and no one would doubt that this story represents the beginning of distinctively modern developments. This was as true of classical science and medicine as it was of classical architecture, literature, or law. Just as Roman law survived into modern codes, so Greco-Roman medicine reached down into recent periods. The writings of Galen, a Greek physician practicing in Rome about 180 A.D., were still authoritative in medical schools when Columbus discovered America more than thirteen hundred years later.

Greek Culture

It used to be said that "Rome was not built in a day." Nor was its whole culture, or that of Greece which preceded it. The origins of both lie in the ancient civilizations of the Near East, whose influence on the early classical world must now be considered. At one time, to be sure, Greek art and science were supposed to have been a spontaneous achievement. But recent excavations have shown that the Hellenes, as the Greeks called themselves, were originally barbaric and borrowed like everyone else from more advanced peoples.

The Hellenes, like the Persians, were an Indo-European people who migrated southward to the civilized regions in or close to the Near East. The former, however, remained largely on the north side of the Mediterranean in the Grecian Peninsula and developed there the first advanced European culture. The chief influence exerted upon the early

Greeks was that of the sea kingdom of Crete. This island was the site of a civilization largely based on that of Egypt and it therefore served as a stepping stone between that land and Greece itself. Unlike the Egyptians, however, the Cretans were a maritime people. They sailed the eastern Mediterranean, in contact with Egypt, Syria, and Asia Minor, and were perhaps the first to realize that this inland sea would in time supersede the Fertile Crescent as the center of civilization. Sea travel made possible wider contacts than Syrians or Babylonians had ever known, hemmed in as the latter were by desert barriers. The Cretan civilization reached its height about 1500 B.C.

Within the next few centuries, Greek invaders conquered the Cretan kingdom and also the coasts of nearby Asia Minor. Ignorant even of writing, the Greeks destroyed much of their predecessors' culture and entered a sort of medieval period of rebuilding. Memories of this era survive in the famous Homeric poems of the Iliad and the Odyssey. These are songs of heroes, particularly of those who fought against the city of Troy in Asia Minor. They reveal early Greek religion as a belief in many gods, the chief of whom was the thunder god, Zeus. The gods dwelt on Mount Olympus in Greece but came frequently to earth to engage in human conflicts. As the Greeks had no earlier literature, these poems became a sort of Bible for them, giving a common literary and religious background and inspiring a traditional opposition to peoples across the sea. Such cultural unity was important because the Greeks—separated by mountain and water barriers into little city-states—always remained politically a divided people.

While winning their struggles against rival cities in Asia Minor, the Greeks gradually constructed their own civilization on the ruins of that left by Crete. In this they were aided by the Phoenicians, another maritime people, whose traders sailed the Mediterranean from their homes on the Syrian coast clear to the Pillars of Hercules (Gibraltar). These merchants brought to Greece the lore of the East as well as that of Egypt.

The most important gift of the Phoenicians was the art of writing and particularly that of writing with an alphabet. Other races of the Near East had long written in signs, each of which stood for a syllable or for an entire word. (This is still true of so-called Chinese characters). But the Phoenicians had modified certain Egyptian signs to form individual letters and this facilitated rapid writing. Their first and second letters, as pronounced in Greek, were alpha and beta—hence we still call the whole list in English the alphabet. The Greeks secured from the Phoenicians Egyptian "papyros," which the Phoenicians called "papyr," whence we get our word "paper." Much of this material came from the city of Byblos, so the Greeks called paper by that name also—much as we term tableware "China" because it once came from that country. And from "Byblos" we get such modern words as "Bible" and "bibliography." Writing with an alphabet on paper was a great improvement over the word-signs on clay or stone which were used in most oriental lands. It provided an essential means for communication in science as well as in literature.

Meanwhile the Greeks gradually absorbed other arts of the East—the use of metals and textiles, and the cultivation of architecture, sculpture and painting. The rudiments of mathematics and medicine were also acquired. Greek artists and scientists in time surpassed their predecessors and a truly Hellenic civilization emerged. By 500 B.C., if not before, the Greeks already displayed the marked originality for which they were ever after so famed. This expressed their independence of mind, an attitude made possible in part by the democratic character of their society. Instead of oriental despotisms, they evolved city governments in which all citizens spoke their thoughts freely. Religious as well as political freedom was finally secured and this had much to do with their intellectual achievements.

The high point of Greek culture was attained in Athens during the fourth century B.C., when that city became one of the most brilliant centers of civilization of all time. There is no space here to follow its political fortunes in the successful defense of Greece against Persian invasions, or in its final defeat by the rival but less cultivated Greek city of Sparta. Nor can the many phases of its life be described. When scholars speak of the beauty of Greek art or of the wisdom of Greek philosophy, they have in mind chiefly the artists and philosophers of Athens. One can only recall here that Athenian culture was spread westward to Italy by Greek trading colonies, and also was carried eastward by the conquests of Alexander the Great. The latter established, about 325 B.C., a great Hellenic empire which reached from Greece to India.

In the course of this dispersion of Hellenic civilization, new centers arose that finally surpassed Athens and other cities of the Greek mainland. In the last three centuries before Christ, during the so-called "Hellenistic Age," beautiful Greek cities were built along the Mediterranean coasts from France to Syria and Greek culture was absorbed by educated men in all these lands. By 300 B.C. distant Syracuse in Sicily was one of the chief Greek cities, and Alexandria in Egypt—named after the Conqueror—was the site of the greatest library and of the most advanced science. It is this latter theme of science, and particularly of medicine, which here merits primary consideration.

Early Greek Medicine

Like other races, the Greeks originally peopled the world about them with demons and spirits and tried to protect themselves by various kinds of magic. Later they learned something of Oriental cults like astrology and so came to believe in more elaborate mysteries. At the same time they evolved the traditions about half-human gods, who fought and loved like men, which have already been mentioned. As might be expected, both folk medicine and magic medicine were practiced side by side, and myths also arose about the relation of particular gods to health and illness. In the Homeric poems, one gets a glimpse of common-sense remedies and of simple wound surgery, of charms against sickness, and of appeals to this god or that to protect a warrior against injury.

The chief healer of Greek mythology was Aesculapius, son of the god Apollo and of a human mother. Being partly divine, he possessed supernatural powers which he devoted to aiding the sick and even to bringing the dead back to life. This enraged Pluto, god of the underworld (Hades), who complained that his realm was becoming depopulated—so many departed souls were being restored to the world of the living. The gods thereupon slew Aesculapius for usurping their control over life and death. But men never forgot what he had done for them and erected little altars to his memory. They also revered his daughters Hygeia (goddess of health) and Panacea (goddess of remedies). It was natural to believe that something of the spirit of Aesculapius and his children lingered about these altars, and people began to come to them in hope of cures. Gradually the altars became shrines, and priests devoted themselves to their care and to that of an increasing number of pilgrims.

In due time a ritual developed, in which those who sought relief first rested and then were purified by baths and ceremonies. Finally they were admitted, usually in the form of a dream, into the presence of the healing god. At the more elaborate shrines like that of Epidairos, beautiful temples, baths, gymnasiums and even theaters were provided. Perhaps the sick, walking in the sunshine or resting above the sea, felt better even before they were admitted to the mysteries. And since they had faith in the ritual, the priests found them willing patients. Many votive tables, left behind by grateful worshippers, testified that the lame had been made to walk and the blind to see. On the other hand, the temples were not always in healthy locations. Hence the supposed cures usually can be ascribed to the fact that many patients recover under any circumstances.

There is no evidence that the temple resorts provided trained attendants. There were women who participated in the mystic ceremonies, as well as priests in charge, but no individuals who could be called nurses. This apparent oversight may be explained in several ways. First, the stay of the pilgrims was not usually a long one. Second, they were not actually bedridden; had they been so, there would have been no way to make the trip from their homes. Nurses are not found today, for that matter, in any formal connection with healing shrines.

Neither Greeks nor Romans, moreover, ever fully understood the value of a nursing personnel. It is true that our own word "nurse" derives from the Latin term "nutrix" (to nourish); but this implied simply a child's nurse and it was only with this concept that the Greeks were familiar. Upper-class families did use slave women as attendants for their children and accorded them honor and affection. But such nurses ordinarily stayed in the nursery.

Beginnings of Science

While the cult of Aesculapius evolved from Greek mythology and provided religious healing, other trends in Greek thought were leading in a quite different direction. The practice of the shrines, however helpful, was but an elaboration of the age-old procedures of priestly medicine. It offered, just as had the Egyptian cult of Imhotep, a blend of natural and supernatural remedies. More novel was the purely naturalistic outlook which was formulated after 600 B.C. in the

Greek cities of Asia Minor. Something of the sort had appeared earlier in Egypt as noted in the preceding chapter, but had taken no permanent hold there. In Greece, in contrast, naturalistic concepts were increasingly accepted by thoughtful men. This trend discouraged supernatural explanations of disease as well as of all other phenomena. Out of this attitude would grow for the first time a completely rational, non-mystical medicine.

Such an outlook, so fundamental to all later science, seems simple enough to us now. Educated persons take it for granted today that the physical world obeys natural laws and that there is no need to give magical explanations of particular occurrences. But this was originally a difficult concept to form, since little was known at first about the relation of one event to the next. As long as natural explanations were unknown, supernatural ones had to be given, for the inquiring human mind demands *some* explanation of everything.

Consider, for example, an eclipse of the sun. When nothing was known of the motions of earth and moon leading up to this, it seemed inexplicable. It was a sudden appearance unrelated to anything that had gone before and could only be interpreted as the interference of an unseen power, of some demon or deity, with the ordinary course of events. (This was still the view of primitive peoples in recent centuries, and European travelers occasionally aroused much awe by foretelling an eclipse from their almanacs and then claiming that they had produced it.) But as soon as the sky paths of earth and moon were measured, it was seen that the latter was bound to get between the earth and sun at a certain time and so produce an eclipse. That is, the moon was bound to do this, *if* its motions always continued to be the same. The only way to see if there was such regularity in the moon's orbit was to keep on observing it, and then to predict at what time it next would be in the eclipse position.

Babylonian astronomers had actually predicted eclipses at a very early period, but they do not seem to have drawn from this any conclusions about natural phenomena in general. About 600 B.C. a Greek philosopher named Thales traveled to Babylon, learned there about astronomical calculations, and upon returning home used these to predict the next eclipse of the sun. Sure enough, the event actually occurred in 585 B.C. just as he had announced it would, and this made a tremendous impression on Greek thinkers. For Thales had made no claims to be a magician who could himself blot out the sun; rather he announced that it all came about inevitably, that it was bound to occur whether or not men cast spells or exorcised demons. Not even the gods had anything to do with it. To foretell eclipses men had only to study the heavenly bodies which could be actually observed; there was no need to look for supernatural forces behind the scenes. To the minds of philosophers, this conclusion banished the gods from the sky-world where Zeus had once ruled.

Thales also visited Egypt, where he observed the majestic pyramids then already some two thousand years old. Evidently the gods had not been wandering on the earth for but a few generations, as Greek myths taught, for here was evidence of a great civilization far more ancient in origin. This seemed to banish the gods from the past as well as from the present. With such thoughts in mind, he and his successors began to study the world about them in purely natural terms. They sought to describe things just as they saw them.

This study of Nature by the philosophers was eventually called "natural philosophy." It was the first clear expression of what we now know as science, which seeks to describe all phenomena as far as these can actually be observed—and no further. Note that science does not solve any of the final mysteries. Thales could tell just when the moon would reach a particular position, but he did not attempt to explain why it revolved or what first set it in motion. Such questions were beyond the scientist and necessarily remained a matter of religious faith or of philosophical opinion.

There were many who distrusted early science. Few knew enough to comprehend it, and it seemed easier to the majority to go on explaining things in a superstitious manner. But philosophers adhered to the ideal of truth for its own sake. They were inspired by intellectual curiosity in a manner which suggests what is now called "pure science." Most of them had little interest in applying ideas or discoveries to useful purposes and they disdained working with their hands. Hence the practical arts were usually left to artisans without benefit of scientific guidance. When, for example, a philosopher discovered the principle of the steam engine some three hundred years before Christ, it was applied only to the making of toys or other trivial devices. In a word, the Greeks contributed much more to basic ideas than they did to technology.

Looking about them, Greek thinkers decided that the world was made up of the four elements earth, air, fire, and water. These substances exhibited, in different combinations, four basic qualities—the hot or cold, the moist or dry. Thus, fire was hot and dry, while water was cold and moist. Everything "under the sun"—rocks, rivers, soils, and even plants and animals—was said to be composed of one or more of these elements. This now seems a naive theory but it reflected the impressions which natural substances first made upon the senses. Later, certain philosophers refined these ideas in relation to more sophisticated problems; as, for example, in advancing an atomic theory about the basic constitution of matter. Meantime, as will be mentioned shortly, they applied their concept of qualities to medical problems in a rather ingenious manner.

Quite apart from theories concerning the ultimate nature of things, philosophers carefully observed the visible forms of various types of natural phenomena—the stars, the surface of the earth, the plants and animals of both air and sea. In this way real sciences of astronomy, geology, and biology were formulated. No less interested in man himself, these thinkers studied accounts of distant lands and invented maps as a means of showing different areas on the earth's surface. They also subjected the customs and institutions of their native cities to a keen scrutiny, and tried to examine the operations of their own minds. Thus emerged the social disciplines of geography, political science, and psychology. Even the forms of human speech, which other peoples seem to have taken for granted, became objects for scientific analysis. Grammar and syntax, for better or for worse, were Greek inventions.

In several of these fields, scientists found it helpful to measure or to calculate—using what today would be called quantitative methods. Unfortunately, they saw little need for this in medicine, and it remained for recent centuries to introduce such methods into medical studies. But in such other fields as astronomy, geography, and the branch of physics known as mechanics, measurements were obviously useful. The Greeks therefore adopted and improved upon Babylonian mathematics. How advanced they became in this respect is indicated, in the case of geography, by their discovery of the global shape of the earth, their estimate of its approximate diameter, and their ability to chart its surface in degrees of latitude and longitude.

45

Here, again, they made little use of these brilliant ideas; and it remained for one Christopher Columbus—some eighteen hundred years later—to make a practical application of Greek geography.

The development of Hellenic science naturally took time. At first only a few philosophers attempted or even understood scientific studies. Then, as Greek cities became wealthy, more of their citizens had the leisure to cultivate learning. Athens, as noted, was the great center of science as well as of art in the days when its trade made it the richest of Greek states. With a population of only about 200,000, it produced during the century following 450 B.C. as many brilliant leaders as any entire nation has done since that time. Here appeared informal schools led by outstanding philosophers like Plato, who taught in a grove called the Academy, and Aristotle, who lectured in a field known as the Lyceum. Plato was interested in mathematics but Aristotle was more concerned with the natural sciences. Alexander the Great, who was a pupil of Aristotle, sent his old master specimens of plants and animals from the lands he conquered and so made his military advance the world's first scientific expedition. Aristotle became one of the great scientists of all time and his writings on physics and biology remained authoritative until recent centuries.

Many present scientific terms come down to us from Greek words of Aristotle's day, since the need of them was then first realized and they were subsequently copied by later Europeans as they became interested in scientific work. From the single word "bios" meaning life, for example, are derived such modern terms as biography, biology, biochemistry, and so on. As we still say, "The Greeks had a word for it."

Medicine, of course, was among the scientific interests cultivated by the Greeks. And in due time it was affected by the transition from a supernatural to a naturalistic outlook on life. While the shrines of Aesculapius continued to offer religious healing, lay physicians accumulated factual knowledge about common illnesses and how to handle them. These men moved from one town to another as skilled artisans and learned much from the bedside. They practiced both general medicine and surgery, and the experience of a number of them was finally incorporated in a collection of writings ascribed to Hippocrates. Although there probably was a physician of that name, he did not write all these works; as his name became legendary, it was applied to the whole collection. This became the first general text on medicine and was long viewed as a sort of Bible by the medical profession.

The Hippocratic texts represent the learning of the chief "school" of Greek physicians, which was originally associated (about 400 B.C.) with Athens and with the island of Cos. Although some theoretical sections now require careful interpretation, the collection as a whole is more modern in tone than anything which had appeared before. The writings relate to nearly all aspects of medicine as we would now envisage them—to hygiene, bedside observations, therapy, surgery, professional ethics, and pathology. Each of these themes, for the sake of clarity, may be considered in turn.

Greek Hygienic Practices

The Greeks, like all men, wished to avoid illness in the first place. The practice of hygiene is more than a medical specialty; it is a way of life which reflects the whole culture of any given society. Now it happened that the Hellenes, like the Egyptians, lived in a semi-tropical region where cleanliness and care in general regimen seemed necessary for the preservation of health. Their esthetic tastes contributed to the same end; filth and carelessness could hardly have appealed to the sense of beauty revealed in their carvings and templed porticos. There is much in the Hippocratic writings concerning diet, the avoidance of sexual excesses, and the importance of exercise. The latter theme reflected the cultivation of physical fitness in the gymnasium. Athletic contests were held regularly, notably in the famous Olympic Games which have been revived during the present century. In Sparta the gymnastic ideal was applied to women as well as to men, and the forms of ideal Grecian bodies have been preserved in masterpieces of sculpture. It should be recalled, however, that all this applied only to the upper classes. Slaves had no time or means to spend on the cultivation of physical perfection.

Greek theories about the spread of disease also contributed to hygienic living. They usually ignored the Jewish concept of contagion in epidemics, and believed rather that disease entered its victims through the air, water, or food which they imbibed. They therefore stressed the dangers inherent in contaminated food and drink or in the breathing of bad air. Experience taught, for instance, that the air

47

in low, damp places was associated with fever and this also seemed true of the atmosphere in places where filth accumulated. Hence they feared bad airs (in Latin, "malaria") and strove to maintain sanitary conditions in their towns. We now understand the partial truth that lay in these conceptions; for malaria really is carried through the air (via mosquitoes) and filthy conditions in a city may be associated with the contamination of water or food. Here was public hygiene, as contrasting with personal, and ideals of this sort were to exert a lasting influence. It is unfortunate that the Greeks did not also appreciate the partial truth that lay in the contagion theory.

Development of Medical Science

Despite all efforts to live in a healthy manner, the Hellenes were naturally subject to disease, and it is at this point that their medicine proper comes into view. Perhaps the best way of introducing this is to recall how their physicians reacted when called to see a sick person: what did they observe and what did they do? Their bedside observations are especially pertinent; first, because they read almost as if written today, and second, because they illustrate well the naturalistic approach to disease which already has been emphasized.

The most striking of the bedside observations are given in a series of case histories, recorded in the Hippocratic book entitled "Of the Epidemics." The account of "Case 1" runs as follows:[6]

> Philiscus, who lived by the Wall, took to bed on the first day of acute fever; he sweated, towards night was uneasy. On the second day all the symptoms were exacerbated. . . . On the third day . . . towards evening, acute fever, with sweating, thirst, tongue parched; passed black urine; night uncomfortable, no sleep; he was delirious on all subjects. . . . On the fifth . . . had a slight trickling of pure blood from the nose; urine varied in character, having floating in it round bodies resembling semen, and scattered, but which did not fall to the bottom; a suppository having been applied, some scanty flatulent matters were passed; night uncomfortable; extremities altogether cold . . . loss of speech, cold sweats, . . . about the middle of the sixth day he died. The respiration throughout, like that of a person recollecting himself, was rare and large, the spleen was swelled upon in a round tumor, the sweats cold throughout, the paroxysms on the even days.

6 Emerson C. Kelly (Ed.), "Hippocrates," *Medical Classics*, vol. 3, William Wood Co., Baltimore (Sept., 1938), 114.

It is hardly necessary to comment on the careful nature of these observations or on how much more complete they are than the brief statements found in Babylonian or Egyptian records. The author of this account recorded all the data that could be secured from general observation, unaided by laboratory devices or instruments. Certain of his phrases are most descriptive. Anyone who has observed so-called "Cheyne-Stokes breathing," for example, will be struck by the phrase "respiration like that of a person recollecting himself."

There are other remarkable things about these histories. In the first place, they are strictly factual accounts. At no point is there the slightest mystery or hocus-pocus. The same attitude, it may be added, is made more explicit in other portions of the writings. This is notably true of the section "On the Sacred Disease" (epilepsy), where magic medicine is consciously repudiated in the following words:[7]

> It is thus with regard to the disease called Sacred: it appears to me to be nowise more sacred than other diseases, but has a natural cause from which it originates like other affections. Men regard its nature and cause as divine from ignorance and wonder. . . . And they who first referred this disease to the Gods, appear to me to have been just such persons as the conjurors . . . and charlatans now are, who give themselves out for being excessively religious, and as knowing more than other people. . . . Its origin is [really] hereditary, like that of other diseases.

Here is plainly a naturalistic view of a mental disorder, a type of illness which was especially apt to be ascribed to gods or demons. Note also the ridicule directed against quacks and the whole repudiation of magic. The statement provides a declaration of independence from all the confusion of folk lore and superstition that had gone before.

Equally impressive is the scientific detachment of these reports. The physician who wrote them was concerned with more than cures; he was interested in disease phenomena as such and in describing them as accurately as possible. More than half of the cases terminated in death, which is noted as calmly as are any of the other data. In other words, the author was a scientific clinician as well as a practitioner.

It was not easy to transcend an interest in the immediate problem

[7] Kelly, "Hippocrates," *Medical Classics*, vol. 3 (November, 1938), 355 ff.

of cures. After all, patients were fellow beings and needed relief. Here was one of the difficulties that doctors always faced; it was hard to view their human data with the detachment that physicists accorded to sticks and stones, or astronomers to the stars. No wonder that for centuries practitioners had concentrated on remedies and given little thought to the underlying problems. Nor would it have afforded much comfort to a dying man, to assure him that an account of his case would aid some later doctor to find a remedy. Clinicians who reported bedside phenomena for their own sake may have seemed cold-blooded to patients and relatives. Indeed, Hippocratic practice has been called merely "a meditation upon death."

This statement is not entirely fair, since Greek physicians did what they could for their patients. Yet even if such criticism had been true, the "meditation" would have been a significant one. Only through these objective accounts of illness could physicians, in the long run, learn much about its nature. The Hippocratic writers thus rose above the human demands of the moment, as well as above magic and superstition. In these respects they anticipated the whole spirit of modern science.

Greek medicine, despite these achievements, was quite different in many ways from modern science. It will be noted in the case cited above, for example, that the account of the illness includes no mention of diagnosis. This would be the first concern of a modern practitioner, who would hesitate to use anything more than palliative treatment until he knew what he was dealing with. But palliative procedures were all that the Greek doctor had at his disposal. And he usually assumed that "the disease" involved was the general condition of the patient rather than any particular entity. The patient shared this view and rarely asked, "*What* have I?" but only "How am I?" and "Will I get well?"

Even when the symptoms described suggest a particular disease to a modern reader, the Hippocratic text is often quite blind to it. Take for example the following notes from "The Epidemics":[8]

> . . . ardent fevers occurred in a few instances; and these
> very mild . . . and never proving fatal. Swellings appeared
> about the ears, in many on either side, and in the greatest
> number on both sides, being unaccompanied by fever so as

[8] Kelly, "Hippocrates," *Medical Classics*, vol. 3 (Sept., 1938), 100 f.

> not to confine the patient to bed. . . . They seized children, adults, and mostly those who were engaged in the exercises of the palestra or the gymnasium, but seldom attacked women. . . . In some instances . . . inflammations with pain seized sometimes one of the testicles, sometimes both. . . . In other respects they were free of disease, so as not to require medical assistance.

This description almost shouts, today, a diagnosis of mumps, but the text goes blandly on without even raising the question of what was involved.

In other words, the concept of a disease entity—separate from but sometimes *in* a patient—was not emphasized by Hippocratic authors. Although they were aware of different "clinical pictures" and discussed the more obvious ones (epilepsy, consumption), they described most illnesses merely as general states of the body. They spoke of fevers and fluxes but made little effort to break these down into specific diseases—hence their indifference to diagnosis.

In contrast, another group of Greek medical writings, that of the "school of Cnidos," did emphasize the existence of many different diseases and the importance of identifying them. But the Hippocratic writers rejected this doctrine, claiming that the Cnidians would confuse matters by naming each and every symptom as a different disease. The Hippocratic view prevailed, and not until some two thousand years later was the doctrine of specific diseases finally revived in modern medicine.

The Nature of Greek Therapy

The Greeks displayed much good sense in treating general states of the body. They related these states to the four basic qualities supposed to be possessed by the four elements. A feverish condition, for example, was hot and dry, and should be treated by substances with the opposite qualities so as to counteract it—that is, by the use of water which was cold and wet. In other words, the feverish patient should have cooling baths and drink plenty of water. Quite the reverse was a common state which we still call a "cold," because the Greeks naturally pictured this condition as cold and wet. And we still follow their logic when we assume that the patient with a cold should be kept warm and dry.

The nature of Greek therapy reflected their general, philosophic

51

outlook. In the first place they were devoted to the ethical principle of "moderation in all things"—medicine included. Secondly, having decided that disease was a purely natural phenomenon, they thought it probable that there were also natural processes of healing. This, indeed, was a matter of common observation. Ergo, the wise doctor simply would cooperate with the healing powers of nature. He should adjust the treatment to the patient's state and also to his individual "constitution." The frail must be handled more gently than the robust.

All this added up, as a rule, to prescriptions of light diets, rest, a few drugs—as laxatives, for example—and of some moderate bleeding. Such practice doubtless did some good, and meanwhile avoided the harm which drastic bleeding, purging, and polypharmacy wrought during many later periods. The Greeks were conscious of their own limitations and practiced a moderation which still commands respect. Note, for example, the aphorism that:[9]

> When things are at the crisis, or when they have just passed it, neither move the bowels, nor make any innovation in the treatment . . . but let things alone.

From long observation, Greek practitioners came to recognize the potential meaning of many clinical signs. They were particularly concerned with an accurate prognosis of the outcome of each illness; partly because this demonstrated their wisdom to onlookers, partly because it was the final outcome which the patient or his friends most wished to know. Even subtle indications of the future course of an illness did not escape attention. Many a modern physician has confirmed, for example, the observation that:[10]

> When, in acute fevers . . . the hands are waved before the face, hunting through empty space, as if gathering bits of straw, picking the nap of the coverlet, or tearing chaff from the wall—all such signs are bad and deadly.

As might be expected from the sane tone of their therapy, Greek surgery was performed with care and restraint. The Hellenes inherited Egyptian surgical instruments and improved upon them in dealing with such emergencies as fistulas, fractures, and amputations. They may also have learned something indirectly from Hindu surgery.

[9] "Aphorisms," in Kelly, op. cit., vol. 3 (Nov., 1938), 301.
[10] "The Book of Prognostics," ibid., vol. 3 (Sept., 1938), 45 f.

Indeed the Hippocratic book "On Surgery" begins by outlining the several elements involved in an operation and then proceeds to give advice on each—much as the Indian classics did in describing medical practice in general. Directions concerning the patient, the operator, the assistants, the instruments and so on, are given in turn. Even such details as the condition of the surgeon's nails are prescribed.

Incisions were made with care and under generally clean conditions. One glimpses procedures that now suggest the need of a nurse. For example:[11]

> The instruments, and when and how they should be prepared, will be treated of afterwards; so that they may not impede the work, and that there may be no difficulty in taking hold of them, with the part of the body which operates. But if another gives them, he must be ready a little before hand, and do as you direct. . . . The bandages should be clean, light, soft, and thin. One should practice rolling with both hands together, and with either separately. . . . That sort of bandaging is the worst which quickly comes off; but those are bad bandages which neither compress nor yet come off.

The Greeks, for all their surgery, never established hospitals. Their operations were performed in homes or on the battle field, much as they would be later in the American colonies. Perhaps their ignorance of the more complicated incisions, even such as the Hindus accomplished, explains the failure to follow the latter in establishing regular institutions of healing. The minor surgery of Greek practitioners, of course, did not demand institutional facilities as much as does major work.

Even in home cases, however, physicians felt the need of more skillful assistants than could be found in the family. Here the Greeks tried an expedient that seems curious in our eyes. This is described in the Hippocratic book "On Decorum" as follows:[12]

> Let one of your pupils be left in charge, to carry out instructions . . . and to administer the treatment. Choose out those who have been already admitted to the mysteries of the art. . . . He is there also to prevent those things escaping notice that happen in the intervals between visits. Never put a lay-

[11] Kelly, *op. cit.*, vol. 3 (Oct., 1938), 163, 165.

[12] For a more free translation of these passages taken from Kelly, *op. cit.*, see John R. Coxe, *Writings of Hippocrates and Galen*, Philadelphia, Lindsay and Blakiston, 1846, p. 78.

> man in charge of anything, otherwise if a mischance occur
> the blame will fall on you.

In other words, students were used instead of trained nurses. This was a part of their apprenticeship, which was the only form of training available before the founding of real medical schools late in the Middle Ages. No doubt the apprentices learned something from this experience and they were presumably more skilled than were members of the family. But one would hardly wish to turn modern cases over to the nursing care of medical students.

Beginning of Medical Ethics

Only men, it is clear, were permitted to study medicine. As in Oriental countries, the women of Greece occupied an inferior social position. Women could not be admitted to the "mysteries" of any art. Hence, even if the Greeks had provided nurses, these would probably have been men. Women did serve as midwives, as in all early lands, but the latter were simply folk practitioners—as they were destined to be until our own time. In other words, a more liberal view of woman's place in society was as much a prerequisite to modern nursing as was the creation of modern surgery or hospitals. It seems strange that the Hellenes, for all their brilliance, never envisaged the possibility that men and women could work as copartners in medicine as in many other phases of life.

Apart from the discrimination against women, which was taken for granted, Hellenic ideals in medical practice were on a high level. A number of Hippocratic books were devoted primarily to the proper conduct of practice. Medicine was viewed as one of the noblest of the arts, though it was admitted that people did not always see it that way. The true physician must be devoted to his profession and to his patients, and must abstain from all actions that could dishonor the one or injure the other. This had already been implied in Hindu classics but was made more explicit in the Greek. In the famous "Hippocratic Oath" the physician swore to labor only for the good of his patients, not to give deadly drugs or produce abortions, to refrain from any improper personal conduct, and to consider confidential such private information as practice might bring him. He also promised not to reveal his art to any save his own sons or other accredited students "according to the law of medicine." This oath is still taken by American physicians, though as a matter of fact it is no longer followed in all respects.

The last provision noted reveals the existence of a self-conscious lay profession, prior to 400 B.C., which sought to control admission to its apprenticeship and then to regulate the conduct of its members thereafter. This guild probably had grown out of earlier secret cults, and continued to hide its knowledge from the laity in order to secure professional prestige and solidarity. Such attitudes were to continue within the profession into modern times. But the greater part of the oath shows a genuine devotion to the interests of the patient and the conviction that this in turn will promote the honor of the practitioner. There is no reference to magic or even to religious sanctions; the medical profession deals only with natural things and stands on its own dignity.

Several of the so-called ethical books provide definite suggestions as to how the doctor should conduct himself. These seem as desirable now as they did more than two thousand years ago, and this explains why Hippocratic ideals have continued to be admired in modern practice. The physician should be careful of his health and appearance, since patients will hardly heed one who is careless about his own body. He should be confident and pleasant in manner but not too gay. At the same time he should be honest about his own limitations, admit uncertainty when necessary, and in such cases request the aid of his colleagues.

When in consultation, doctors should avoid bitter arguments and disputes. They should be fair to one another as well as to their clientele. They are even reminded that mediocre practitioners "get by" simply because most illness is mild or self-limited—just as a poor sailor gets along well enough in fair weather. But as the real test for the latter comes with a storm, so the doctor has his trial in desperate cases. It is for this that the good doctor must prepare himself—modestly, earnestly, and without pretense. Here, in the effort to reconcile the best interests of patients and practitioners, was the basis of a sound professional ethics.

Evolution of Pathological Concepts

All the aspects of Greek medicine so far discussed—clinical observations, therapy and surgery, and the ethics of practitioners—relate to obviously practical matters. There was, in addition, a theoretical side to Greek medical thought which influenced practice at the time and which would dominate later medical thinking for many centuries. Since they had inquiring as well as observant minds, Hellenic physicians were not content simply to observe and treat their patients; they also desired to know what really went on, or "went wrong," in the bodies of sick persons. The symptoms they observed were apparently signs of inner and mysterious changes, and if the nature of these changes could be discovered they could be dealt with more intelligently in practice.

In other words, the Greeks became interested in the study of disease processes, and they had to think about these in terms of such knowledge of anatomy and physiology as they possessed. Being the first to pursue this science of disease, they gave it a name. The word "pathology" comes from Greek "pathos" (suffering), plus another term "ologia" (to speak); that is, pathology literally means "to speak of suffering."

Unfortunately, symptoms rarely gave any good clue as to what lay behind them within the body. Exceptional were the skin diseases, where superficial sores seemed in themselves to be the main pathological process. But most illnesses displayed a confused picture, with certain common symptoms—fever, pain, rapid pulse, headache, and so on—recurring in various combinations. Such behavior patterns frequently related to more than one part at a time. The patient "sick of a fever," for example, might simultaneously exhibit intestinal disorders and all the other signs just mentioned. Moreover, even one symptom such as fever or rapid pulse could be felt in every part at the same time. The natural conclusion was that in most of these cases something had gone wrong throughout the entire body. What could this generalized pathological process be?

It was very difficult to find an answer. Greek physicians could not see inside their patients, as they had no instruments with which to aid vision or to reach inaccessible parts. They were not well informed about the normal behavior of organs, to say nothing of the abnormal. Little could be learned in physiology without experimentation; and for some reason not easily explained, Greek scientists rarely realized the value of that procedure. This may have resulted in part from their disdain for manual labor which was left to slaves. To experiment would have required the use of the hands and physicians may have considered this beneath them. Be that as it may, they depended largely on simple observation of whatever Nature happened to show them.

This procedure worked well enough in a field like anatomy. Greek physicians acquired a fair knowledge of gross anatomical structures from a dissection of animals. But when it came to explaining how these structures worked in life, passive observation could reveal little and that little was often confusing. Thus, when the Greeks observed mental processes, these seemed to be associated with the heart rather than the brain. This was especially true in the case of the emotions. Did not the heart beat faster with either hope or fear? We still speak as though this Greek view were true; for example, we refer to "a heart-felt need" or to "affairs of the heart," despite the fact that we know this organ has little to do with such emotional experiences.

How confused Greek notions of physiology were, despite their knowledge of anatomy, can be illustrated by the following quotation from the Hippocratic text "On the Sacred Disease." The author seeks to explain why the victim of epilepsy becomes speechless and froths at the mouth; that is, he attempts here to envisage pathological physiology:[13]

> The man becomes speechless when the phlegm, suddenly descending into the veins, shuts out the air, and does not admit it either to the brain or to the vena cava, or to the ventricles, but interrupts the inspiration. For when a person draws in air . . . the breath (pneuma) goes first to the brain . . . and part to the veins, and from them it is distributed to the other parts of the body along the veins; and whatever passes to the stomach cools and does nothing more; and also with regard to the lungs. But the air which enters the veins is of use (to the body) by entering the brain and its ventricles, and thus it imparts sensibility and motion to all the members, so that when the veins are excluded from the air by the phlegm and do not receive it, the man loses his speech and intellect . . . and the eyes are distorted owing to the veins being excluded from the air; and they palpitate; and froth from the lungs issues from the mouth. For when the breath does not find entrance to him, he foams and stutters like a dying person.

It is plain here that the Greeks had little understanding of either

[13] Kelly, "Hippocrates," *Medical Classics*, vol. 3 (Nov., 1938), 361 f.

the respiratory or circulatory systems. The "phlegm," which is the villain of this drama, was supposed to originate in the brain, an idea that may have been based on observing mucus descending in the nostrils during a cold. From the brain, this phlegm "suddenly descended" into the veins to work all the havoc noted.

Ordinarily the Hippocratic physician did not get as close as this to a specific account of what went wrong in a given illness. Since he usually thought in terms of some condition common to the whole body, he sought rather for some equally generalized pathological process. Now just what was so widely distributed throughout the organism that any abnormality therein would produce simultaneous disturbances in various parts? There were at least two possible answers. First, there were certain fluids or "humors" that permeated many parts, notably the blood and (they believed) the phlegm and bile. And it had long been known that the blood and probably the other fluids were vital to the preservation of life; ergo, anything abnormal in them would be dangerous to the whole body.

From such observations the Greeks derived their classic "humoral pathology." This was the doctrine that most illness was due to some derangement in the fluids, either because impurities had gained access to them or because they were out of proportion one with another. Most important were the famous four: blood, phlegm, black bile, and yellow bile, which were supposed to correspond to the four elements of air, water, earth, and fire. Blood was said to originate in the heart, phlegm in the brain, yellow bile in the liver, and black bile in the spleen. If a man was ill, it was believed that this was caused by such conditions as impure blood, excess secretion of bile, or "a sudden descent" of phlegm from the brain as described above.

On such a basis the Greeks also constructed a sort of psychology. A man's temperament depended upon the "humor" which happened to be dominant in him. If it were the blood, he was said to be "sanguine"; if the phlegm, he was called "phlegmatic"; if the bile, he was "melancholic"; and these terms continue to be used now much as they were originally employed.

Lacking real evidence regarding pathological processes, this was about as intelligent reasoning as the Greeks of 400 B.C. could employ. They made the best of common experience and then pieced it out with speculation concerning what might be the case. Nor was there anything wrong with such speculation in itself. It seemed sensible to blame things on the blood and clinicians would still agree there was some truth in this. Modern conceptions of "blood poisoning" or about the role of hormones fit approximately into the old humoral picture. The trouble was that there was no way of checking the truth of the theory by further observation or experiment. Hippocratic writers had no way of finding out whether blood or bile actually was impure or out of proportion. Only instruments and experimentation, both of which were lacking, could have made this possible. The Greeks just assumed all this to be true because it was plausible and because they wanted some theoretical framework on which to hang their intrepretation and practice. They took a speculative short-cut, across fields of unrecognized complexity, to a theory that seemed to explain everything. They had no idea of how little they really knew about disease processes.

One of the attractive things about the humoral pathology was that it seemed to explain all illness by a single cause (state of the fluids), and hence suggested a single type of treatment. Obviously this was to be found in one or more methods of getting rid of impure or excess fluids, in the hope that Nature then would replace these by normal supplies. One could eliminate the humors by bleeding and purging. These age-old procedures now were encouraged further by this theoretical justification.

The Hippocratic reliance on Nature tended to keep bleeding and purging in bounds; but in later times these would be carried to extremes and other elimination devices such as sweating thrown in for good measure. So recently were these heroic methods in vogue that they still survive in folk practice, which absorbs ideas from regular medicine slowly and then retains them after the latter has abandoned them and passed on. Some Americans believe to this day that if they "catch cold," they should immediately swallow a purgative, take hot drinks and baths, cover themselves with quilts and so "sweat it out of them." Nor is it long since a dose of sulphur and molasses was taken in the spring, in an annual attempt to "purify the blood." So the shadow of Hippocrates lingers over thousands who have never so much as heard his name.

Although the humoral pathology always remained the most popular in classical medicine, one other major theory was advanced.

There was a second possible answer to the question, "What is so wide-spread in the body as to explain the simultaneous appearance of symptoms throughout?" In addition to the fluids, there were anatomical systems of solid parts, blood vessels and nerves, which also ramified everywhere. It was therefore just as plausible to assume that illness might be due to a disturbance of these systems. Eventually a school of thought developed which ascribed all disease to an excessive tension or to an equally excessive laxity in the blood vessels or in the nervous system. Such a current conception as "high blood pressure" is a partly analogous idea.

Those who accepted this view, clearly formulated by Greek physicians in Rome about 125 B.C., were known as Methodists—not to be confused with the present religious denomination. Theirs was a "solidistic," as contrasted with a humoral pathology, and was referred to in Latin phrase as the *strictum et laxum* theory. They spoke much of "the right tone" in vessels or nerves and sought treatments which would promote this if it were lacking. That which would restore tone eventually became known as a "tonic." While Hippocratic doctors trusted the healing powers of Nature, Methodists believed in a more vigorous interference with Nature. Yet the possible dangers of such interference were more potential than real, since Greeks were restrained in practice by the ideal of "moderation in all things."

It does not seem to have occurred to the disciples of either of these schools that there might be some truth in each. Humoralists could see no good in Methodists and vice versa. It is now known of course that disease processes involve both the fluid and solid parts. But theorists were so anxious to have one, beautifully simple explanation of everything, that they would not complicate it by looking for truth outside. This is what might be called the "either-or" fallacy in reasoning and it was destined to confuse medical thought down into recent times.

In addition to being one-sided, speculative theories about pathology tended in time to inhibit further investigation of the nature of disease. If the cause of all sickness was thought to be just one factor such as the condition of the humors (a monistic pathology) and this led to just one form of treatment like fluid elimination (a monistic therapeutics), there seemed to be little more to be discovered. Bleeding or purging, along with a sensible regimen, were supposed to be good for everything; what more did anyone need to know? Palliative drugs might be found from time to time but this would not change the general picture. So reasoned generations of later physicians, who were content to assume that all necessary knowledge was at hand. In a word, monistic pathological ideas, intended originally to enlighten physicians, became eventually an obstacle to medical progress.

There were some Greco-Roman physicians who sensed this danger and who therefore rejected pathological theories altogether. But since they themselves had no scheme to follow, they depended simply on a trial-and-error search for remedies and hence were known as "empirics." Such men were scorned by the theorists as being little better than folk practitioners, and the phrase "a mere empiric" came to mean a complete ignoramus in medicine.

Meantime, one can now see, the path to real progress lay midway between speculation on the one hand and groping empiricism on the other. The philosophers were correct in claiming that theories were important and the empirics were right in urging the observation of facts. But these two approaches needed to be brought together, so that theories could provide clues for seeking significant facts and the latter in turn would verify or refute the theories. Otherwise, speculation remained "up in the air," while facts about remedies were assembled helter-skelter and without meaning.

The Origin of Medical Research

This rational way to medical progress was briefly envisaged by a number of Greek physicians of Alexandria, who shared the benefits of that great cultural center. Unlike other medical men up to that time, they were supported by the state and so did not have to devote all their time to practice. Nor did they need to fear public prejudices. Officials permitted them to dissect human bodies, in order to secure anatomical knowledge and also to search at autopsies for evidence concerning particular illnesses. It is even said, though this is doubtful, that they practiced vivisection on condemned criminals. Uninhibited by popular needs or taboos, this Alexandrian group undertook the first studies which today would be termed "medical research."

The primary advances made were in the science of anatomy. Thus Herophilus, who was active about 300 B.C., gave more accurate accounts of human structures than had ever been available in the Hippocratic literature. He was able, for example, to distinguish between tendons and nerves which had looked so much alike to early observers; and he determined that the brain was the central organ of the nervous system and the nerves the carriers of sensation. He did not, however, recognize abnormal conditions in organs and simply accepted the usual humoral pathology.

More remarkable in this respect was Erasistratus, who flourished during the following generation. Knowing how organs ordinarily appeared, he found in post mortem examinations that they were sometimes changed by disease. If a man died of "dropsy," a vague symptom complex, the liver was found to be hard; but if death followed snake bite, this organ was soft. Illness might then be something more than a corruption of the humors; perhaps it was a process that went on in the organs themselves. This view had something in common with that of the Methodists, in that it related disease to the solid parts of the body. But the Methodists thought only of a generalized tension throughout whole systems like the blood vessels; whereas Erasistratus now envisaged disease as a process which went on in a particular part. This conception of a localized pathology was eventually to prove of great value.

In its cold-blooded objectivity, Alexandrian research was analogous to that of the Hippocratic clinicians whose case histories have been quoted. Just as the clinicians reported the behavior of bodies during illness, the Greco-Egyptian group recorded the condition of bodies after death—the other side of the picture. Neither at that time, nor for long periods thereafter, did there seem to be much connection between such clinical reports on the one hand and pathological findings on the other. Perhaps this can be ascribed to the fact that both lines of investigation were begun only to be abandoned shortly thereafter. Neither was carried far enough to bring out the mutual relationship involved. No one saw, for example, that the cough observed in "consumption" at the bedside might be correlated with tubercles found in the lungs at autopsy.

Both clinical and pathological studies were subsequently discouraged for reasons that were largely social and professional in nature. Many of the necessary ideas were available by 300 B.C., but there was no social soil in which they could flourish. Bedside practitioners were too busy treating patients to make careful reports on them; the forty-two case records from which quotations were given above are unique in the whole medical literature until modern times. The Alexandrians were more free, as noted, to do detached work, but their findings were largely ignored because they were of no immediate use in practice. Erasistratus, indeed, was ridiculed as a mere theorist because his discoveries seemed to have no practical value. Had Greco-Roman society been familiar with printing and had medical journals been available, Erasistratus might have spread his views so widely that they could not have been forgotten. But all these things lay far in the future. Meanwhile, the university and library at Alexandria lost governmental support after Cleopatra, the last of the local rulers, was defeated by the Romans in 30 B.C. Pure research declined thereafter in the one classical center that had really encouraged it.

Only in recent centuries have the two paths of investigation, the clinical and the pathological, been brought together so as to permit the identification of diseases that cannot be recognized by bedside observation alone. It is true that the Greeks, even if their society had encouraged it, might not have been able to accomplish this because of their lack of necessary instruments and procedures. Their indifference to experimentation would have handicapped them, even if all professional facilities had been available. One can summarize the whole story by saying that in their ideas the Greeks anticipated modern medicine but failed to develop it because of both social and technical limitations. How modern physicians finally overcame these difficulties will be the theme of later chapters.

Chapter IV

Imperial Rome:

Greek Medicine, Roman Administration, and
Christian Idealism

The Greek city states, which had once defended themselves successfully against the Persians, eventually lost their independence to Rome, a new power in the west. Italy had remained a primitive land of stone-age culture until after 1500 B.C. About that time, the Indo-European migrations which had sent waves of people into India, Persia, and Greece, also involved a movement of Italian herdsmen across the Balkans and down into their long peninsula. They came in such numbers as to give their name to the entire region, although they did not hold all the area at first occupied. Their villages in northern Italy were overrun after 1200 B.C. by Etruscan invaders, a race apparently expelled from Asia Minor by the early Greeks. And in southern Italy the Italian tribesmen were dominated by Greek colonies, whose cities flourished there and in Sicily throughout the Hellenistic Age.

During the ninth and eighth centuries B.C., the Etruscans, who had brought an oriental civilization with them to the west, established flourishing cities throughout northern Italy. About 750 B.C. one of their princes conquered the Italian village of Rome on the banks of the Tiber. Under Etruscan rule the Romans absorbed new arts, for example, the use of bronze. They also acquired a written language and skill in the construction of stone buildings. Later they learned much from the cultivated Greeks to the south, but the basis of their civilization remained Etruscan with Greek refinements superimposed thereon.

An illustration of Etruscan influence can be seen in the Roman use of the round arch. The Greeks rarely, if ever, employed this form. But the Etruscans had acquired the idea from Persia, brought it with them to northern Italy and so passed it on to Rome whence it eventually spread throughout Western Europe. Hence the ancestry of such round-arch buildings as the Roman Colosseum, or of early medieval cathedrals, runs back via the Etruscans to the temples of the ancient Near East. This is worth noting because of the common misapprehension that all Roman culture came directly from Greece.

About 500 B.C., when the Greek cities were entering their most flourishing stage, Rome overthrew its Etruscan rulers and entered a period of growing power that was finally to make it master of the Western World. The people of the city had remained largely Italian in blood and Latin in language. With the aid of related Latin tribes, Rome gradually acquired control of central Italy, and passed from a simple farming community to a thriving commercial center. In the course of trading with Syracuse and other Greek cities in the south, the Romans acquired the Greek alphabet and adapted it to the Latin tongue whence it has come down to us in the modern European languages. There were, of course, many other borrowings. First the Romans took over the tangible things of Greek culture—money, textiles, sailing ships—but later they absorbed ideas as well. Greek art, religion and, last but not least, science finally seeped into the Roman way of thought.

This is not to say that the majority of Romans ever came to think just as did the Hellenes. The usual opinion is that the Romans were a less brilliant people, and their arts and sciences have been considered mere continuations of the Greek. In medicine, as will be noted, they copied and organized but do not seem to have been highly original. On the other hand, this view can be exaggerated. In engineering and other kinds of technology, the Romans far surpassed their predecessors. They copied Athenian temples, but they also constructed great roads, aqueducts, and types of public buildings of which the Athenians never dreamed.

The citizens of "the Eternal City" also displayed an administrative genius which enabled them to both conquer and organize a lasting empire, whereas the Greeks could not long maintain even a union of local allies. Originality can express itself in law and government as well as in speculation, and Roman law has survived almost as long as Grecian philosophy. Modern peoples are in most respects closer to the Romans than to the Athenians; and the administration of at least one present institution, the Roman Catholic Church, has come down directly from Roman origins.

Roman Government

While absorbing much from the Etruscan and the Hellenic civilizations, the Romans were developing their own government along original lines. This became republican in form, with popular assemblies, a senate, and several executives called consuls. In times of emergency, temporary dictators were appointed. Meanwhile, disciplined, professional armies (legions) were developed, as well as an efficient navy. Such military power grew during a series of wars that Rome fought with rival powers in the western Mediterranean area. Her chief opponents were Carthage on the African coast—originally a Phoenician colony in the West—and the Greek cities of Sicily. The latter were overthrown by 275 B.C., and Carthage was finally destroyed in 145 B.C.

Such expansion was made possible in part by the concentration of power in the hands of one man. As wars occurred in more distant regions, it became harder for a large body like the Senate to direct them and there was need for a single executive. Meantime, the increasing wealth of the city made ambitious consuls anxious to seize such power. There were bitter contests between them, from which Julius Caesar first emerged victorious after his conquest of Gaul. Caesar was about to make himself permanent dictator, when he was assassinated by those devoted to the old republican government (as told in Shakespeare's play "Julius Caesar"). His place was then secured by his heir Octavian, later called Augustus, who became the first dictator-emperor. Augustus controlled the legions and it was their support which enabled him and his successors to rule. In due time the Senate gave him the titles of "princeps" (literally "the first" citizen), and "imperator" (meaning a commander). He and his successors also took

Caesar's name as a title in itself. From these terms are derived such modern titles, respectively, as prince, emperor, and "Kaiser" or "Czar."

Augustus and the emperors who followed him were dictators in fact if not in title. Sometimes they named their own successors, sometimes the throne was seized by military leaders. As in all such systems, the government worked well when the emperor happened to be able and just. But when he was incompetent or cruel, as in the cases of Nero and Caligula, the people suffered. Those who know the book or moving picture called "Quo Vadis" will recall the story of Nero, who took sadistic delight in the torture of his many victims and yet was deified as the emperor of the greatest domain in the world.

Until 180 A.D. most of the emperors were able leaders, and it was during these first two centuries after Christ that the high tide of Roman civilization was attained. Rome itself became a city of about a million people, with magnificent buildings and a complex society. Similar but smaller towns flourished throughout the provinces from Britain to Africa, and from Spain to Syria. (A Roman coastal town, Pompeii, can still be seen much as it was about 75 A.D.; since it was then submerged by ashes from the nearby volcano of Vesuvius and was never uncovered again until almost 1800.) Peace was maintained by the professional legions. These troops also enforced the famous Roman law, which eventually provided a large measure of justice. This law became more humane as time passed. Women and children were protected from possible cruelty, and women were given such other rights as control over their own property. Even slaves were given a certain degree of protection. Needless to say, the arts flourished under these happy circumstances and there was some cultivation of Greek science in both Greece and Rome.

Unfortunately, from 180 A.D. to almost 290 A.D., the throne was seized by a series of military adventurers termed the "barrack emperors." There actually were eighty rulers in the course of ninety years! Some of this disorder was due to economic difficulties but it was increased by the lack of firm and enlightened government. Weaknesses appeared which no outward grandeur could conceal. Wealthy men secured most of the lands in Italy and elsewhere; and the former farmers either became serfs on great estates (villas) or drifted into towns where they depended upon the government for "bread and games." Thus, while agriculture declined, city life became debased and the population began to fall. It became difficult to find good soldiers in Italy and the legions enlisted undisciplined barbarians instead. Meanwhile, the Germans outside the Empire pressed across the frontier, and in the East a new Persian kingdom (Parthia) revived to harass the Romans in that region. By 280 A.D. it looked as though the Empire might go to pieces because of decay within and pressure without.

This catastrophe was averted by a new line of strong emperors, beginning with Diocletian in 284 and ending with Theodosius about 400 A.D. But their control was only made possible by a complete oriental despotism, in which all vestiges of the freedom of citizens and of the old republican forms disappeared. These last emperors divided the realm between two capitals, Rome in the West and Constantinople (Istanbul) in the East. Internal decay continued, and gradually the military power was so weakened that masses of Germans filtered in across the Rhine and Danube and took up lands within the Empire. The Emperor Constantine moved the capital from Rome to the eastern city which bore his name and Italy became a mere province. The West was left relatively unprotected and after 400 it was submerged by a series of Germanic invasions.

Emergence of Christianity

It was Constantine who became the first Christian emperor. Long before his time, however, the old Roman religion had declined and its place had been taken by various Oriental cults. When the Christians first appeared, they were viewed only as an obscure sect of Jews who were bringing in another religion from the East. Many of them were martyred during Nero's reign, chiefly because they would not join in the religion of the State and worship the Caesars. Gradually, however, more and more people found in Christianity a hope for which they had long been groping. Dangers and disillusionment, which many experienced in a decaying Empire, led them to a faith which preached brotherhood in this world and salvation in the next (Roman religion had held out no prospect of a blessed hereafter). The poor and humble, in particular, found in the Gospel a greater promise than was contained in all the edicts of man-made gods.

The original accounts of the life of Jesus had been written in Aramaic, the Syrian language which He actually spoke. Greek accounts were later prepared, and four of these—the Four Gospels—were eventually combined with the epistles of Saint Paul and certain other writings to form the New Testament. This, together with the Jewish Old Testament, became the Bible of the Christians. Inspired by these writings and by the example of the martyrs, Christianity spread steadily despite government persecution. At first it was an underground movement. Indeed, it was literally underground, for there are still miles of catacombs under Rome where early Christians hid their worship and buried their dead. The converts organized churches which they called by the Greek word "ecclesia" (assemblies), whence comes our word "ecclesiastical."

While the Roman government was declining in energy and power, these churches became more vigorous. The morale of their members seemed to improve with persecution. Finally the emperors, faced by constant invasions from without the Empire, no longer could struggle against this growing influence within. In 311 A.D. an edict granted Christianity the same rights as other religions, and somewhat later it became the official faith of the Empire.

The Christian Church promptly became a well organized and active institution which was destined to outlive the Roman State. Those most active in the service of the churches became the clergy, and their leaders in the cities became bishops who had religious authority over surrounding areas known as "dioceses." Under Roman civil administration, numbers of dioceses were combined to form a province; and following this system, the Christians set up archbishops to direct the churches throughout an entire province like Spain or Gaul. Among archbishops the most influential was the Bishop of Rome, whom Catholics believe was granted divine authority to rule over the entire Church. The bishops of the East, however, reflecting the division of the Empire, refused to accept the authority of the Bishop of Rome. This in time led to a division between the Roman and the Greek Orthodox churches.

During the last century of the Western Empire, while the government was crumbling, able men turned more and more from business or political careers to the service of the Church. Whatever happened to the Empire, the new religion would survive and would spread to all peoples, barbarians and Romans alike. Many of the German tribes were indeed Christianized before they crossed the borders and this eased the shock of their invasions. The Church carried on and eventually became the only institution common to all parts of Western Europe. It therefore bridged the medieval gap between classical and modern times, preserving something of ancient culture until this could be revived nearly a thousand years later.

Roman Medicine

During their more prosperous periods, the Romans took over and maintained the Greek tradition in science; but they added little that was original save in technology. Indeed, right through the Roman era, many artists and scientists continued to be Greeks who worked in Athens or Alexandria, or who at times came to Rome. Nothing done by Romans equaled the earlier astronomy of Ptolemy of Alexandria, who viewed the earth as the center of the solar system; or the physics of Archimedes of Syracuse, who discovered the principles of the lever in mechanics. Nor did Roman mathematicians advance beyond Euclid's geometry. Strangely enough, the Greeks had never invented a good system of notation and the Romans also lacked imagination in this respect. The latter continued to use clumsy "Roman numerals" which we now employ only for formal purposes. As a result, they did not evolve an effective arithmetic and did their ordinary figuring on counting boards. One can easily understand this difficulty, if he will try to do any simple example in Roman figures; for instance:

$$IX \times XLIII = ?$$

This lack of modern arithmetic, which was more difficult to develop than was geometry, was a handicap to both business and science throughout the classical and medieval periods.

The medicine of the Romans, prior to their contacts with the Greeks, involved the usual mixtures of folk, magical, and religious practices. Even after these contacts, the practical Italians were suspicious of Greek refinements in art and science and were inclined to view Alexandrian medical research as so much "high falutin' nonsense." As Rome and other cities grew, however, the demand for medical advice increased, and all sorts of practitioners appeared in shops offering infallible remedies or mystic balms. We would now call these individuals quacks or charlatans but such terms imply a contrast with a "regular" profession. As there were no such regular physicians in early Rome, there was nothing illegal about this quacking chorus with its refrain of "good for what ails you." Medical practice was simply a free-for-all.

As early as about 200 B.C., shortly after the conquest of Sicily, a few Greek physicians moved thence into Rome. They were at first viewed with suspicion but gradually their superiority to local quacks became evident to upper-class Romans. Here was a native practitioner who obviously had had no special training but who claimed to have found some universal remedy. Could he compare with a Greek who had been trained in a "school," that is, who had read the Hippocratic writings under the guidance of older physicians and had taken a solemn oath admitting him to a dignified guild?

After 100 B.C., Greek physicians were admitted to citizenship. This gave them much needed protection in the courts and some of them acquired fame and fortune. In the later days of the Empire, while political and military power declined, the position of physicians continued to improve. Government support was given to medical instruction and some attempt was made to license educated practitioners so as to distinguish them from quacks. There is evidence that women practiced in this period, though relatively little is known about them. Municipal doctors were appointed to care for the poor without charge. These arrangements concerning "medical police" were largely abandoned in the Middle Ages and then revived in recent centuries.

The improved position of physicians reflected increasing respect for a regular, educated tradition in medicine. This attitude also expressed itself in the fees and social prestige of those who acquired a fashionable practice. Galen, a Greek practicing in Rome, is known to have received as much as several thousand dollars in a single case. But this does not mean that ordinary practice was in reputable hands. Most practitioners made their money by bleeding slaves or selling love philters, while quackery of all kinds continued to flourish. The minority of well-informed physicians was always handicapped by competition with the ignorant and unscrupulous. This situation persisted almost to the present time.

Another handicap faced by Roman medicine was the lack of encouragement for original investigations. Prestige depended on personal practice or official position, rather than on a reputation for research. Although the later emperors gave some support to professional education, they established no real medical schools and eventually abandoned the University at Alexandria. Romans were a practical folk and wanted immediate cures, rather than basic research that might prove of use in some distant future. They were inventive enough to work out "shorthand" writing but never thought of a printing press. With no printing, there were no journals which might have strengthened the position of reputable doctors. Last but not least, the few who attempted original work found their way blocked by the old aversion to human dissection. It is one of the curiosities of history that the same Romans who enjoyed seeing living men torn by beasts in the arena, did not allow the dissection of dead bodies for scientific purposes. Their sensitive souls could not tolerate the sacrilege.

It is not surprising, under these circumstances, that the course of Roman medicine was largely a continuation of trends already observed in the Greek. There were the same theoretical systems of pathology and practice, the same controversies between humoralists, solidists ("Methodists"), and empiricists. The saving grace in all this was, as before, the "moderation in all things" so emphasized in the Hippocratic Writings. In the best days of the Empire, down to about 200 A.D., a number of distinguished Greeks and Romans did carry Alexandrian research a little further, and pointed the way which would have led to real progress if only any number had followed it.

One of the most remarkable of these medical authorities was Celsus, a Roman, whose works were written about 25 A.D. He prepared an entire encyclopedia, of which only the medical section survives. His work was largely ignored by contemporary medical men, perhaps because Celsus was not a physician himself, and it was forgotten during the Middle Ages. Celsus recognized the importance of medical history and we owe to him most of what is now known of Alexandrian medicine. He was also the first to translate Greek medical terms into Latin—the form in which they are now usually employed. Celsus recognized the importance of basic research, had some opportunity for animal dissections, and as a result advanced beyond Greek anatomical knowledge. It is evident, for example, that he understood the real function of arteries, which had hitherto been thought to carry only air.

One of the most significant aspects of Roman medicine, as revealed in Celsus and other writers, was the field of hygiene. They inherited and maintained the Greek ideal of a sound mind in a sound body (*Mens sana in corpore sano*). Since their outlook on life was a practical and worldly one, the upper classes appreciated the advantages of health and beauty. They made a cult of cleanliness and the other physical virtues, at the same time viewing disease with repugnance and showing little sympathy for its victims. With wealth and leisure, to be sure, came various dissipations; but an account of such evils at the courts of corrupt emperors should not be taken for a picture of society as a whole. Perhaps more serious was the tendency to commercialize sports in the arena, and to admire physical vigor in the gladiators rather than to develop it in one's own person. Like the Greeks, moreover, the Romans made physical perfection an ideal only for the upper classes. Working people had no time for such a luxury.

In harmony with their devotion to individual health, the aristocracy developed a remarkable régime of public hygiene. They accepted the Greek view that diseases spread largely through contaminated airs and waters, and then applied this conception with their usual administrative and engineering skill. The location of camps and towns was carefully chosen to assure good air, usually on high, dry ground to avoid *malarias*. Public works were constructed to secure supplies of pure water for both bathing and drinking purposes. Great aqueducts running for hundreds of miles brought mountain streams to the major cities, and some of these are still standing. Rome provided more water per capita than did any modern metropolis until recent decades. Much of this supply was used in the public baths, which served as general club houses for the comfortable classes. Vestiges of these *thermae* survived in medieval villages and also have come down to us in so-called Turkish or Russian baths.

Systems of sewers, of course, had to be constructed in order to provide both drainage and sewerage facilities. One sewer constructed in Rome several hundred years before Christ, the *cloaca maxima*, is still in use. In imperial days, the city possessed more than fifty public latrines—a figure which compares favorably with most American communities at the present time.

Unfortunately, the other side of this picture was an indifference to the Jewish concept of contagion in the spread of diseases. While not entirely unknown, it was given little attention. Hence Roman neglect of isolation procedures was as marked as was their emphasis upon sanitary control. The results were what might be anticipated from modern knowledge. Where diseases were due to conditions in the air or water supply, as in the case of malaria or typhoid, they were long checked in Roman towns. But where diseases were spread by contact, there was no control. Terrible epidemics, as of bubonic plague, swept the Mediterranean world at intervals. The decadence of later days, moreover, witnessed a decline of even sanitary administration. Malaria became a menace, and certain historians have blamed this disease for the final "decline and fall" of the Western Empire.

Roman Hospitals

The practical genius of the Romans expressed itself in surgery, as well as in sanitary engineering. The surgical work described in Celsus, for instance, shows technical advances beyond Hippocratic practice. Notable was the use of the ligature in operations. Celsus mentions more than a hundred instruments—scalpels (Latin, *scalpri*), forceps (Latin, *forceps*), and so on—and most of these have actually been found at Pompeii just as they were described. One would expect surgical progress among a military people like the Romans. But even with them, this art remained largely devoted to emergencies and superficial incisions. Their theories of fluid pathology did not indicate any need for operations upon hidden, solid parts. Perhaps for this reason, also, there was no demand for the hospitalization of ordinary patients. Minor operations could be done in homes or in the booths of physicians.

Hospitals were provided, however, for two special classes. One of these was the military group. The legions were necessarily away from home and so needed places where they could be given medical care. Motivated partly by this situation, the Romans evolved a regular system of military hospitals. Here their administrative genius came into play again. They might not have ideas as original in medical theory as those of the Greeks, but they could plan and build an institution more effectively. A few years ago, several of the original military hospitals of about 100 A.D. were unearthed in the Rhine and Danube valleys. As such border areas had to be constantly defended against barbarians, these buildings probably served as base hospitals for frontier forces. The ground plans reveal long corridors from which opened a series of suites—each of the latter containing two private rooms connected by a small hall. In addition there were central courts for kitchens, dining rooms, pharmacies, and so on. Apparently there were no wards, so it may be assumed that each soldier-patient enjoyed considerable privacy. Many surgical instruments have been found in the ruins, indicating that advanced Roman wound-surgery was here placed at the service of the troops.

Presumably, either slaves or soldiers detailed for the purpose acted as orderlies—the type of service which was still depended upon in military hospitals at the beginning of the American Civil War in 1861. It is known that each legion had its medical officers and no doubt some of these were stationed in the base hospitals. Despite the lack of trained nurses, the whole scheme of these oldest known hospital buildings suggests careful planning in the interests of the sick and wounded men.

Such planning, however, is not to be ascribed to humanitarian motives. Soldiers were essential to military power and so had to be given the best of care. Similar hospitals were also provided for slaves on large estates, where again a selfish motive—in this case the desire to preserve one's own property—was involved. On the other hand, no hospitals were provided for the poor or for the population at large, since here there was no immediate advantage to be gained by their construction. Only a more humane attitude toward the sick at large could inspire the building of general hospitals, and it was this attitude that Christianity first infused into the Roman world in the fourth century. It is conceivable that the institutions for soldiers and slaves provided administrative models, which the Christians later followed in providing service for all who were in need.

Christian Influence on the Development of Humanitarian Concepts

No one will deny that Christ taught a distinctly humanitarian religion. The first and great commandment was to love God, and the second "to love thy neighbor as thyself." The parable of the "Good Samaritan," so totally different in spirit from the usual Roman indifference to suffering, must have made a marked impression on early Christians. True, other religions in the empire expressed high moral ideals. There was the Stoic code of the Emperor Marcus Aurelius, for example, which taught men to rise above their sufferings and from which we derive the adjective "stoical." But the best of the pagan philosophies lacked that sincere concern for the poor and humble, that warm sense of universal brotherhood, which was so distinguishing a feature of Christianity.

Christ even identified the love of one's neighbors with the love of God, in His promise that "inasmuch as ye have done unto the least of these my brethren, ye have done it unto me." Moreover, He definitely stressed the care of the sick, not only in his own works, but in such statements as: "I was sick and ye visited me." Illness was thereby made an object of special consideration, rather than of repugnance and disdain. In like manner nursing was lifted above the level of drudgery to a plane of moral and religious obligation. Among Christians it immediately became a respected occupation, in which the most unpleasant work was ennobled by a sense of devotion to a great cause.

Most active in such service were the women of the new faith. Perhaps this was because women had been accustomed to tend members of their own families in illness, if servants were not available, and now projected this work beyond the family circle. Perhaps they were more inclined to compassion than were the majority of men. In any case, Christ's teachings tended to place men and women on an equal plane and this encouraged the public activity of the latter in charitable undertakings. Leadership was naturally assumed by women of means who could afford the time and expense of aiding numbers of patients. Since the social position of upper-class women had improved in the later Empire, they had acquired control over their own persons and property and were in a position to devote themselves to charitable endeavors. In point of general equality with men, the position of women was better in the third and fourth centuries than it was to be again until the last hundred years.

In outlining the circumstances which brought women into nursing after 300 A.D., at least three factors must therefore be noted: first, the improvement in the social position of Roman women; second, the Christian teaching of the equality of men and women before God—and therefore in God's work; and, third, the Christian appeal to carry on His work in behalf of all who were in distress. When women actually served as nurses in homes or hospitals, they presumably employed Greek concepts in medicine along with Roman experience in hospital administration. Thus the heritage of hospital nursing involved a synthesis of Greek medicine, Roman institutions, and Christian ideals.

There are several references in the New Testament which suggest that certain women, even in the earliest Christian communities, devoted themselves to those in need. Thus St. Paul refers (*Romans,* XVI, 1) to "Phebe our sister" who "hath been a succourer of many and of myself also." It is true that during the two following centuries, there is almost no record of such women. But their activities must have expanded meanwhile, for after 300 A.D. there are many references to so-called deaconesses (from the Greek *diakonoin,* to serve or to minister) who devoted themselves to serving others. Their duties may have at first been largely religious, but visits to homes doubtless involved them in nursing activities when the need became apparent. By 400 A.D., about the time of the fall of the Western Empire, the Deaconesses had acquired dignity and influence in the Eastern churches. They were apparently ordained as a clerical group and worked in close association with the bishops, but little is known about their actual nursing activities. Similar groups of women were at times referred to as "Widows" or "Virgins," but these titles again afford little information as to their actual labors.

In the Western or Roman church, deaconesses were rarely mentioned; and their ordination was forbidden by Church Councils after 400. But St. Jerome has left clear accounts of women who carried on good works in the Rome of that period. Notable were a group of wealthy lay patrons like Marcella, who organized a community of charitable women which had something of the form of later convents. Probably the most famous of these ladies was Fabiola, who has been viewed almost as the patron saint of early nursing and whose idealized portrait is so well known. She erected what is sometimes called the first hospital in Rome and nursed patients there with her own hands.

It is not to be supposed, however, that the construction of early Christian hospitals was left primarily to the charity of individual women. If the deaconesses of the early Church helped those in distress, this was probably done in homes or in relief stations something like modern Salvation Army units. This aid related no more to nursing than to any other type of service. After the Church was openly established, the bishops also felt responsible for expanding charitable facilities. Hence one hears in the fourth century of "houses" for the sick, for strangers, for the poor, and for the aged. (We still speak of "poorhouses.") Usually it seemed more economical to gather all classes of unfortunates into one institution known as a *xenodocheion*, which was the ancestor of the modern hospital as well as of most other types of charitable institutions.

As the bishops came to have funds and power, they built permanent institutions of this type. As early as the Council of Nicaea, which formulated the Nicaean creed in 325, it was decided that each bishop ought to establish a *xenodocheion*. A few of these were apparently founded in the Eastern Church during Constantine's reign and they became more common there in the fifth century. In the Western Church also, bishops seem to have been responsible for the earliest institutions for the poor; although Fabiola, as noted, is said to have built the first real hospital during the fourth century. St. Jerome, in describing the latter, used the Greek term *nosokomeion* (house for the sick) rather than the Latin term *hospitalia* (for a guest), and this suggests that the idea of a hospital was still novel in Rome and so he had to employ a Greek word for it. It was not until the sixth and seventh centuries that references to any such institutions became frequent in Western Europe. In Gaul the Frankish King Childebert established (540) a hospital at Lyons, which exists to this day and which is probably the oldest in the world.

Little is known of the nursing service which was provided in these hospitals of late Roman days. At times deaconesses may have served as nurses, perhaps under the direction of a wealthy patron. Eventually nursing orders were formed in the Church to serve in hospitals, but this was a later development to be noted in the next chapter. Meanwhile, it is quite likely that servants did most of the ordinary labor under the direction of Church authorities. There is no suggestion that these folk, some of whom were probably women, received anything more than rule-of-thumb training.

In like manner, there is little knowledge of the medical services available. There was, to begin with, a revival of faith healing. It was natural for Christians to appeal, in their sufferings, for divine aid. Perhaps this was especially so in an age when ordinary medicine could do so little for the sick. No one who has prayed for the recovery of a patient given up by physicians should be unable to appreciate this.

But in the course of the Middle Ages, amidst general ignorance, religious healing often became a matter of charms which were reminiscent of magic medicine. And healing shrines were sometimes suggestive of the temples of Aesculapius or of other ancient cults.

Early Christians seemed at times distinctly hostile to classical science. One can understand that, after long persecution, they felt an aversion to certain aspects of Roman culture—to its religions, sports, and even in some degree to its arts and sciences. Christian and pagan ideals would have clashed in any case, however, because of basic divergences. Even the best of the pre-Christian Romans were primarily interested in *this* world; they had a secular orientation. Christians, in contrast, centered their aspirations on the next world; they had a religious and somewhat ascetic outlook. Good men, they held, would cultivate the spirit which was eternal rather than the pleasures of a body which was carnal and perishable.

Some of the leaders of the Eastern Church carried this asceticism to extremes. They isolated themselves as hermits so as to deny themselves any worldly pleasures whatever. St. Simeon Stilites actually lived on the top of a pillar for many years, to the admiration of all who beheld this paragon of self-denial. Some later religious orders, even in the West, also despised the body as the source of temptation and sought to "mortify the flesh" in order to establish the victory of the spirit. Their members, who were celibates, were urged never to bathe and to eat only the coarsest food. Such attitudes hardly encouraged personal hygiene or the employment of medical science. There were instances in which Christians were disciplined for even studying pagan medicine. This very word "pagan," which was applied to everything non-Christian, still conveys unpleasant associations.

It would be a mistake, however, to overdraw this picture. The ascetic practices of hermits or of a few monastic groups were not typical of the great majority of the clergy or laity. There was no general abandonment of worldly affairs with the triumph of Christianity, although the more brutal aspects of public life—such as the sports of the arena—were usually suppressed. Normal economic and cultural activities continued in Roman cities, save where these were submerged by barbaric invasions. Any general objection to taking over pagan arts and sciences was eventually answered by the doctrine of "the spoils of the Egyptians." This was the view that, just as the Israelites had been able to filter out the finer things in Egyptian culture, so the Christians could save the worth-while aspects of Roman life and discard the baser elements. Hence Roman temples were taken over as Christian Churches, and Roman medical advice was probably employed in early Christian hospitals. Even though the human body was not to be cultivated for its own sake, it could still be viewed as the temple of the spirit and was therefore not to be unnecessarily injured or neglected.

Decline of Science

Although the extent to which the early Church opposed classical science may have been exaggerated, the fact remains that this science was declining. Sporadic medical research came to an end after about 200 A.D., and the standards of practice slowly deteriorated. Two factors largely explain these trends; first, the limitations inherent in Roman medicine itself and, second, those imposed upon it by the barbarian invasions from without.

As has been observed, Roman medicine was never noted for originality. Research had been the work of a few individuals like Celsus, who kept alive the best of the Greek tradition. But the mass of practitioners did nothing to advance medical science, and desired only some handy "system" which they could apply indiscriminately to daily practice. This desire to have everything worked out was natural enough. Busy doctors at the present time like to have one general text which sums up the whole field of practice, or even briefer handbooks which abstract all that is needed in a particular field. Such attitudes are not inconsistent with good practice today, because research centers keep pouring new knowledge into revised editions of these texts. But since no research centers were supported in Rome, there was no source for revisions, and there was constant danger that some comprehensive system would be finally accepted as a permanent guide to practice. This was exactly what happened to the teachings of the Greco-Roman physician Galen, whose work was so impressive that no basic attempt to improve upon it was made for more than a thousand years after his time.

Galen was a well-educated Greek who came to Rome for fame and fortune during the latter part of the second century. He acquired a fashionable practice and exercised wide professional influence. He was an original observer and even something of an experimenter. He performed physiological experiments as well as ordinary dissections upon animals; for example, he severed the spinal cord at different levels in order to demonstrate its functions.

Galen's goal was to prepare a complete account of all medical fields and then to tie it all together in a system which could be used as a final guide. Lawyers did this sort of thing in legal codes, why could doctors not do likewise? Now the only way to systematize medical knowledge was in terms of some theory of pathology, since the central problem was necessarily the nature of disease. All inquiries in medicine led ultimately to the basic question: "What happens in the sick body?"

Unfortunately, Galen lacked any real knowledge of pathology and so had to speculate about disease processes. And he could think of no better hypothesis than that inherited from the Hippocratic literature; namely, that illness results from the condition of the body fluids or humors. He knew of different clinical pictures like consumption or the skin diseases but assumed that these were mere expressions of underlying, humoral conditions. In a word, this Greek physician held that the nature of all disease was known and that there was little need to search for distinct disorders. Nor was there any urge to find specific treatments, since only humoral depletion by bleeding or purging was required.

In a word, Galen had all the answers. In his last years he wrote:[14]

> I have continued my practice on until old age, and never as yet have I gone astray whether in treatment or in prognosis, as have so many other doctors of great reputation. If anyone wishes to gain fame through these, and not through clever talk, *all that he needs is, without more ado, to accept what I have been able to establish. . . .*

A modern physician who made such claims would be considered a fool or a charlatan, and this contrast suggests the vast difference between the medicine of 200 A.D. and that of our own time. Galen's successors, unhappily, took his word for all this. Hence his system, which dominated medicine in the late Empire, actually discouraged further research. There was nothing more to discover!

14 Quoted in Henry E. Sigerist, *The Great Doctors*, New York, W. W. Norton and Company, Inc., 1933, p. 76

Tendencies inherent in Roman medicine were thus making for decadence, long before Christianity became dominant in the Empire. This decline in science was a phase of the general deterioration of Roman civilization after the second century. Then the infiltration of barbarians into the Western Empire after 400 A.D., brought about an actual disintegration of Roman culture during the so-called "Dark Ages." Medicine and all the sciences were involved in this catastrophe. The Church alone, of Roman institutions, survived intact, and the clergy became the only educated persons. Struggling to preserve the remnants of classical arts and sciences, and not always well trained themselves, the best these clerics could do was to pass on something of Roman medicine as they had received it. It was unthinkable, under the circumstances, that they could improve upon such writings as those of Galen.

Meanwhile, the Church continued to build hospitals in its effort to meet the needs of the poor, and the deterioration of medicine inevitably expressed itself in these institutions. The lay medical profession declined and almost disappeared, so that hospitals soon had to depend upon priests for such medical service as the latter could provide. Since medicine could only be an avocation with the clergy, the future of medical science looked dark indeed.

One may sum up by saying that the Church carried over into the Middle Ages a heritage of hospitals which was a great humanitarian achievement. On the other hand, these institutions displayed no scientific interests; in part because of the religious preoccupations of their directors but more because of the decadence of medicine in a backward age. The medieval period was to witness a flowering of Christian idealism in hospital nursing, but this nursing was to be handicapped by a serious lack of medical guidance.

Chapter V

The Middle Ages:

Medicine and Nursing in a Christian World

In 410 A.D. a migrating German group, the Visigoths, captured and plundered the city of Rome. Such a catastrophe had not occurred in centuries, and it seemed to Roman leaders that civilization was going to pieces before their eyes. Historians, sharing this view, used to date the fall of the Empire and the beginning of the "Dark Ages" from that year. Actually, the disintegration of Roman culture was a long process; it began before 410 and continued for centuries thereafter. There is no need to review here all the migrations, wars, and political upheavals that disturbed these centuries. Many of the changes were destructive, and there is no question that the early medieval civilization which followed was inferior to that of the Classical age. Yet some constructive trends also appeared in time, and out of these would emerge the beginnings of modern culture and society. Something should therefore be said of the more general aspects of medieval history.

There were two main periods of barbarian invasion. The first, from about 400 to 700 A.D., saw various German tribes overrun the Western Empire. Their home lands had been east of the Rhine and north of the Danube; but Slavic and Mongol peoples attacked them from the East, and this in turn forced the Germans over the Roman frontier along those rivers. Most important were the Goths, who conquered northern Italy; the Franks, who conquered Gaul and gave their name to that land (France); and the Angles and Saxons who descended upon Britain, after whom that country came to be known as Angleland (England).

All of these peoples had a similar background. They had the virtues and defects of a hardy, primitive people. Their men, who devoted themselves to hunting and to war, were at times violent and disorderly. They and their families were organized into small tribes which followed the leadership of local chieftains. Although familiar with simple agriculture and with decorative arts, they were entirely illiterate. They naturally impressed the Roman gentry as being ignorant and brutal. In a word, the early Germans never had developed so high a culture as had, for example, the Indians of Mexico and of Peru.

It was long customary to view the barbarian invasions as having been purely destructive. Naturally there was much in Roman life that the newcomers could not maintain. Sometimes it was worse than that. The Anglo-Saxons who conquered Britain had had no contact with Christianity and simply wiped out Classical culture there for the time being. Except for those who fled into Wales, the original Britons were either destroyed or absorbed into the Anglo-Saxon population. Latin customs and speech entirely disappeared; and as a result the language and law of England (and therefore of the United States) became and still is basically Germanic.

On the other hand, more of Roman culture survived near the center of the Western Empire in Italy, Spain, and Gaul. The invading tribes in these areas were already Christians and their penetration was something like that of rough and illiterate immigrants. Unused to commerce or manufacturing, they left the cities to decay and settled as farmers on the old estates. Trade and communication declined, and law and order were maintained uncertainly by local leaders. But these barbarians had some awe for the traditions of the Empire and loyalty for the Church. Hence Roman institutions survived in modified forms. We still refer to modern Italy, Spain, and France as "Latin countries" and say that they speak "Romance languages."

After they had had time to settle down, German leaders temporarily established large kingdoms like that of the Franks in Gaul. The greatest of the Frankish leaders, Charlemagne, even tried to revive the Western Empire, and did succeed for a few years in reuniting France, Germany, and Italy into what he called the "Holy Roman

Empire" (800 A.D.). He and his German successors claimed, clear down to the nineteenth century, to be the heirs of the Caesars. All this, however, was but the shadow of the old Empire in the West. Soon after Charlemagne's death his heirs quarreled, and France, Germany, and Italy fell apart—never to be united again.

Meanwhile the Eastern Roman Empire carried on, and maintained a modified Greco-Roman culture until Constantinople was finally captured by the Turks about 1450. This so-called Byzantine government had no control over the West. Moreover, both Constantinople and the remnants of Charlemagne's Empire were soon threatened by another danger from the Near East. A prophet named Mohammed appeared in Arabia and his followers began to spread his religion by the sword. They worshipped Jehovah and their sacred book, the Koran, was similar in some ways to the Old Testament. But since they denied the divinity of Christ and were viewed by the Christians as infidels, the two religions came into sharp conflict. Between about 630 and 730, the Mohammedans conquered Persia, Syria, and northern Africa, and threatened to spread into Europe. The Eastern Emperor stopped them at Constantinople; but in the West they overran Spain and were checked only when they invaded France. They held parts of Spain throughout the Middle Ages, and to this day the culture of North Africa and of the Near East is primarily Mohammedan (Moslem) in character.

After Charlemagne's death, therefore, the old Roman Empire was permanently divided into several regions dominated by different peoples and different civilizations. A remnant of the Eastern Empire persisted in Constantinople and in the surrounding territory. Here art and science were maintained on a higher level than in the West, though not with the vigor of Roman days. In the Near East, in Africa, and in Spain, Moslem culture flourished. The Mohammedans absorbed Roman civilization and added to it in some ways with great success. They were particularly apt in maintaining Greco-Roman science, and were later to return this learning to Europe after it had almost disappeared therein. Finally there was Western Europe, divided politically between the remnants of Charlemagne's Empire but united in religion by the Church centered in Rome. This region became, between 800 and 1100, the most divided and the most backward of all the areas mentioned; yet it contained the formative elements of modern civilization and therefore deserves primary consideration.

Development of Feudalism and Monastic Orders

Charlemagne's Empire, as noted, was only a shadowy one. Tribal leaders, who became known as nobles or lords, held local control over their followers. After trade had broken down, travel was no longer safe and most people lived in rural isolation. These conditions were accentuated by a second series of barbarian invasions that broke out after 800. This time it was the Vikings, Scandinavian folk as yet untouched by Christianity, who overran the half-civilized German peoples already within the old Empire. Descending from Denmark or Norway, Viking sea-raiders spread terror from the Baltic shores clear around to the Mediterranean. In Britain, in France, and in Sicily, they looted and destroyed, spreading terror and forcing each community to defend itself as best it could.

Under these circumstances, the efforts of Frankish or other German leaders to rebuild kingdoms and to restore Roman government largely broke down. Instead, a form of society evolved which was known as feudalism. Political, economic, and social life were all based on the holding of land. The typical social unit became the rural manor, owned by a lord with his castle on the hill and worked by peasant farmers who lived in hovels in the village below. The latter had to raise food for the lord as well as themselves and were bound to the soil as serfs. They could not be sold away as slaves, however, and the lord was expected to protect them against outside foes. The lord, in turn, sought further protection by swearing allegiance to some more powerful nobleman and promised to fight for him when necessary. The descendants of Charlemagne, or those who usurped their places, were still called kings, but became in fact simply local lords themselves. Government was a matter of hundreds of petty principalities, united only by the vague allegiance owed by small lords to greater ones.

The only institution which transcended this confusion was the Church, which maintained throughout Western Europe an organization paralleling that of the old Empire. The pope's position was analogous to that of an emperor, while archbishops and bishops were in charge of smaller areas. The basic ecclesiastical unit was the village parish, in charge of a "secular" priest. Outside of all this organization, save for the final authority of the pope, were the "regular clergy" of the monastic orders. More will be said of them below.

In theory, the Church was absolute in religious matters but left civil affairs to feudal lords. In practice, however, it was difficult to separate the two fields. Bishops often became landlords themselves, and the pope held control of the Papal States around Rome as a civil ruler. The Church had its own courts and controlled many matters, such as education and family law, which are now to a large degree in the hands of the State. Under these circumstances, the Church and feudal lords sometimes came into conflict and the former for a while became supreme.

In the early Middle Ages there were only three large classes in society. The mass of the people were serfs, ignorant farmers living under primitive conditions and bound to the soil. Above them were the aristocratic and warlike lords. Finally there were the clergy—secular and monastic—who stood somewhat apart from the other groups. Although bishops might become nobles, their powers were not hereditary like those of ordinary lords, and even poor men might improve their lot by entering the services of the Church. Celibacy was required of both the secular and regular clergy in order to secure an undivided devotion to the religious life, and this also tended to make churchmen a group apart.

Careers in religious orders were open to women as well as to men. At a time when most women had again fallen into a subordinate position, it was possible for others to acquire dignity as nuns and for gifted individuals to become leaders of regular communities. There were even joint monasteries of men and women, living in separate houses but ruled over by a woman superior. Certain of the orders, both for men and for women, came to devote themselves to nursing; and it was this trend that brought women into such service for the first time on a large scale. By the modern period, indeed, nursing began to be viewed as primarily a woman's field.

The advent of monastic institutions in the late Roman Empire has already been noted. As medieval life became increasingly dangerous, more men and women who were spiritually-minded yearned to escape from worldly chaos. Others, less devoted, doubtless entered monasteries for security and protection. In the Eastern Empire communities tended to be extremely ascetic and to remove as far as possible from all interests save spiritual contemplation. In the Western Church, however, monastic groups often devoted themselves to good works; that is they established communities of celibate brothers or sisters devoted to a religious life but working to maintain themselves and also to aid the poor folk about them. They were "in the world but not of it."

Perhaps the best illustration of this is to be found in the Benedictine order. St. Benedict, a wealthy Roman born about 480, established at Monte Cassino a group of strictly disciplined monks. He gave them a famous "rule" which became a model for many later orders. This required all members, after a year's probation, to vow never to return to the world, to give complete obedience to their leader (abbot), and to deny self by humility and service. To avoid temptation, the monks must devote their time to worship and to work. Benedictine monasteries spread throughout the Western Church and, wherever established, became of great value to local communities. The monks, being disciplined and intelligent, became the best farmers and also kept alive a little of the Roman skill in handicrafts and manufacturing. They produced enough to sell and so kept trade from dying altogether.

In like manner, the monks kept alive the vestiges of learning. Since they continued to use the Roman language (Latin) in religious services, they had to be educated in that language and so could read surviving Roman classics in art and science. The brothers copied these old manuscripts and it was in this way that some knowledge of the past was preserved. The bishops, meantime, established cathedral schools which carried on similar work; and certain of these schools finally evolved after 1200 into the first European universities. Notable among the latter were Oxford, Paris, and Bologna. Originally composed of unorganized scholars, these bodies secured charters that made them independent of local bishops or lords and enabled them to pursue learning in a systematic fashion. In due time, they established the earliest faculties in theology, in law, and—with one exception—in medicine.

Following the Viking invasions, some two centuries were required before European life again became stabilized. One is dealing here with long periods, when great changes could occur even if these went on slowly. When a man of Charlemagne's time (800) looked back to the "fall of Rome" (410), it was across a longer interval than we now scan in recalling the Pilgrim Fathers at Plymouth. And at the height of medieval civilization (about 1250), a similarly long interval was involved in looking back to Charlemagne's time.

During the later Middle Ages, conflicts between rival lords continued to disturb life but other forces provided for progress. In the eleventh century, for example, certain inventions improved agriculture and this slowly raised the living standard of the masses. Notable were the invention of the horseshoe and of a better form of harness. These have long since been taken for granted but they made possible the first systematic use of horses on farms. Hence they were really labor-saving devices, analogous to the McCormick reaper of the last century. Medieval peoples pioneered in seeking such devices, perhaps because Christianity had encouraged humane attitudes toward labor. (Ancient societies had depended upon slaves and usually did not feel any need for easing their burdens.) Perhaps also there was some shortage of workers in medieval Europe and this likewise encouraged labor-saving inventions.

While agriculture slowly advanced, there was a parallel improvement in urban life. As surplus products became available, trade picked up and towns took on new life. In them there again appeared a "middle class" of merchants, artisans, and shopkeepers; that is, a class which in social standing ranked midway between lordly nobles and lowly serfs. These townspeople or burghers resented the power of landed aristocrats. They used money in trade, and this enabled them to employ soldiers and to become independent of the nobility. Eventually the middle classes sided with monarchs, in overthrowing the feudal lords and in establishing modern kingdoms.

Manufacturing revived within the towns as trade and transportation improved. Ideas were exchanged and new devices introduced more rapidly in urban centers than on rural manors. Skilled workmen developed the arts of working in textiles, in metal, and in glass. All this was done by hand, but ingenious machinery was invented to use water, wind, or animal power—as in water wheels, windmills, and treadmills—to aid the hand-workers. One notices here, again, the desire to save human labor. The chief artisans had their own shops, and organized guilds of master-workers to control competition and to insure the quality of their products. Apprentices were admitted by a guild to learn the trade. They then became journeymen who worked for others, until they could complete a "masterpiece" and be admitted as guild members with shops of their own.

These master-workmen made possible the flowering of medieval art after about 1100. Metal workers made armor for the nobility which, both in beauty and in strength, surpassed the best equipment of the old legions. Stone masons produced the great medieval cathedrals, architecturally more intricate than any buildings Romans had ever reared. Indeed, architecture attained to new heights, literally and figuratively, after 1200. In this age the Romanesque style, employing heavy walls and round arches, was superseded by the Gothic with its high walls, pointed arches and towering spires.

Christian idealism found expression in these Gothic forms. One need only stand before a great Gothic church today to feel again something of this medieval aspiration. To the aid of architecture, the Church also brought the associated crafts of sculpture and of stained glass. Another art, music, was transformed by adding to the old elements of melody and rhythm the new conceptions of harmony and counterpoint. Musical notation or writing was invented for this purpose. There can be no doubt that the later Middle Ages was one of the great periods in the history of art.

Medieval skills had meaning for medicine as well as for manufacturing and art. Thus, glass makers were able, by the thirteenth century, to make lenses that slightly improved vision—the first spectacles. This idea of an instrument to aid the senses had never occurred to Classical peoples and it had great import for the future. Four centuries later, lens-grinders would finally make the first microscopes and telescopes, and the use of instruments of this sort would become a basic factor in modern science.

Not all improvements in arts and crafts were due to native ingenuity. Much was gained by reviving contact with Constantinople. Indeed, Eastern Europe—modern Russia—derived the beginnings of its civilization directly from the Byzantine Empire. Hence the Greek alphabet and the Greek Orthodox Church survive there to the present time. But more was gained by Western Europe through contacts with the Moslem world in Syria, Africa, and Spain. The famous crusades, in which Christian forces tried to wrest control of the Holy Land from "the infidels," finally failed in that object. But those who fought in these wars brought back superior Moslem products and this had a stimulating influence on the West. It proved more profitable to trade with Mohammedans than to fight them, and considerably more healthy.

Commerce slowly revived in the Mediterranean, bringing superior Oriental steel, leather, and textiles into Italian ports whence they were distributed to northern countries. Some of these materials, like Oriental rugs, maintain their fine reputation to the present time. Especially prized were new foods and drugs, such as the spices of the East Indies. Often the Europeans named new goods after the lands from which they came and these names still reveal the far reaches of this early trade. Thus, "damask" cloth came from Damascus, "cordovan leather" from Cordova in Spain, and "China" ware from the distant land of that name. As Oriental goods were distributed through Western Europe, the process stimulated trade and so provided some further improvement in living standards.

Tangible goods were not the only imports from the East. There were also ideas. Persian art may have had its influence on Gothic cathedrals. But most important was the impact of Arabic science. At all points where Western scholars were in contact with Moslem thinkers—notably in southern Italy and in Spain—Christians were stimulated to take up the almost forgotten scientific interests of the Roman period. This theme calls for a brief consideration of medieval science and particularly of medieval medicine.

Status of Science

The early Germans, as did other races, cherished beliefs in gods and demons. In English, because of our Teutonic background, we still name certain days of the week after these old gods—as in Thursday for "Thor's Day." Christianity replaced the folk religion but many superstitions survived. Among the more pleasant ones that still persist are the belief in the magic power of mistletoe and some of the customs associated with Christmas. Descendants of the Roman peoples also clung to their belief in magic and the whole cultural decline of the early Middle Ages encouraged this outlook on life. Among the ancient beliefs which took on new vigor was Babylonian astrology, which flourished until the seventeenth century. Because this was quasi-scientific, with its study of the stars, it was readily absorbed even by learned men and medieval science was saturated with it. As noted before, there are still persons who time their medical treatments by the phases of the moon and others who indulge in the hocus-pocus of horoscopes.

Another quasi-scientific discipline was the study of alchemy. This was directed toward the discovery of the "philosopher's stone" which would turn base metals into gold, or toward a search for "the fountain of youth." The Arabs brought alchemy into Europe, as the name implies. ("Al" is the Arabic definite article, and one finds it in other scientific terms owed to the Moslems; for instance, algebra, alcohol, alkaline, and so on.) The medieval alchemist seemed half wizard, half scientist, for in his search for magic powers he had to pry into the nature of all materials. So he mixed and boiled and evaporated everything—metals, alkalies, acids—that came to hand. In this way he learned something by trial and error, and his mysterious den became the first chemical laboratory. Perhaps unknowingly, he developed the experimental method which the Greeks had never fully appreciated. This method, like the use of instruments of observation, was to become a basic factor in modern science. When churchmen and others revived classical science, however, they tended to despise alchemists as magicians and so ignored the experimental procedures that might have done much for research. Only after 1600 would the alchemist's methods become respectable and make possible the present study of chemistry.

Roman knowledge of mathematics and the physical sciences barely survived after 800 in the monastic copies of old manuscripts. Much indeed was lost. But after 1100, Arabic translations of Greek originals were brought into Western Europe and these revived interest in the writings of Aristotle and of other Greek scientists. Learned scholars of the thirteenth century, like Albertus Magnus, knew the physics of Aristotle and the geography of Strabo. The last-named work revived the Greek idea of the globe, which was later to be helpful to Columbus.

Probably the most significant contribution of Arabic science was an improved mathematics. Borrowing from India, the Arabs had developed basic number signs (digits) running from 1 to 9, and added the symbol 0. The latter seems an ordinary idea now but was a remarkable invention at the time. Who could have first thought of a sign which stood for simply nothing at all! Europeans had never had a word for the conception and so we still call it by the Arabic term "zero." Using the symbols from 0 to 9, numbers could then be written with place values in terms of tens, hundreds, and so on. Thus, "240" really means two hundreds, plus four tens, plus no digits. Immediately a more effective arithmetic became possible. Compare the simplicity of multiplying 240 by 21 in these "Arabic numerals," with the difficulty of doing the same example in Roman numerals. The new arithmetic was first useful to business men but was eventually of great aid in all the sciences.

Hence one may say that the three basic methods that finally made modern science possible—the use of experimentation, of instruments of observation, and of mathematical procedures—all had their beginnings largely in the Middle Ages. The subsequent revival of Greek science, with its emphasis on passive observation, had its value; but without these newer methods, modern science would never have so surpassed the best efforts of Classical days. This fact should be remembered when the superstition and the ignorance of medieval science are described.

On the other hand, only the germs of the newer methods, so to speak, could be observed in that period. Their value was potential rather than actual. Only the alchemists did much experimenting, no microscopes were yet available, and even physics was more a matter of theorizing than of measurements. There was great awe for Classical authorities in all fields, and a tacit assumption that it was impossible to improve upon them. The best minds gave most of their time to theology rather than to Nature, for final truths about God and man seemed more important than did natural surroundings. The schoolmen of the universities did sometimes assert that reason was a better guide than "authority"; but in their debates about this they emphasized logic rather than actual observation of the world around them.

Here and there an original scholar like Roger Bacon began to take notes on natural phenomena and even to talk about experimentation. He appreciated the importance of mathematics and had a great faith in the future wonders that science would perform. Notable were his apparent predictions of flying machines, self-moving vehicles, and x-rays. But he also believed in astrology, and like his contemporaries was blind to modern distinctions between the natural and the occult.

In such an intellectual atmosphere most scientific discussions were settled by citing an earlier authority or by long and subtle arguments. Such "scholastic" procedures are still employed to some extent in law, where cases are settled in part by citing the decisions of earlier judges and by elaborate arguments between opposing counsel. It is now hard to realize that medical matters were once determined in the same way. Like modern lawyers, all that most medieval doctors needed in their investigations were the immediate evidence (patients' symptoms) and a good library.

Revival of Classical Medicine

The medicine of so long a period as the Middle Ages cannot be described in any simple, uniform manner. Roman and German superstitions, Christian faith healing, surviving Classical science, and practical experience were all combined in varying proportions according to the particular time and place. By selecting the right sources, the story can be made one of hopeless ignorance or, conversely, one of some progress. These were "dark ages," but there were also gleams of light amidst the darkness.

During the fifth and sixth centuries something of Roman medicine survived, particularly in Italy and France. For a time, the majority of physicians continued to be laymen. It was in this period that some religious leaders opposed secular medicine as "pagan," and offered instead the hope of miraculous cures. This was sometimes done frankly on the ground that secular medicine had failed them—which was no doubt true. Thus Gregory, Bishop of Tours, relates that:[15]

> I had suffered so much [from dysentery] that I had no hope of life. The doctor's antidotes were absolutely ineffective. In desperation I called Armentarius the royal physician and said to him: "You have tried every expedient of your art and your drugs are of no avail. One thing remains. I shall show you a marvelous cure. Take dust from the sepulchre of St. Martin and make a drink from it. . . ." After taking this drink my pain was eased and I recovered my health.

After about 600 A.D., with the further decline of civilization in general, only priests seem to have maintained medical practice in Northern Europe. Although lacking medical training, priests had some learning

[15] Quoted in Loren C. MacKinney, *Early Medieval Medicine,* Baltimore, Johns Hopkins Press, 1937, p. 67.

and so could be set above folk practitioners and quacks. The more complicated Greek works were too much for the clergy, but they compiled Latin summaries of medical writings which were helpful in every-day practice. Emphasis gradually shifted after 900 A.D. to this naturalistic medicine, as contrasted with magic or miraculous healing, although the latter elements persisted into modern times.

Ordinary monastic practice absorbed considerable folk medicine and was therefore less harmful than the elaborate procedures of later centuries. Thus, the Abbot Strabo put his ninth-century compendium of remedies in a poetical form easily remembered. He used only simple drugs, as when recommending the value of the humble radish:[16]

> A piece of this hot-flavored root bitten off
> And chewed, will expel the most shattering cough.

Nor was he entirely lacking in the folk virtue of humor, as the following extract testifies:

> Again if your stepmother bears you ill will
> And mixes a poisonous aconite pill
> In your food, and rejoices to see you look sad,
> As you swallow the drug and begin to feel bad
> Never worry, but drink of a cup of this herb,
> Your stepmother's evil designs it will curb.

During the later Middle Ages several influences brought about a decline in so-called monkish medicine. With the rise of universities, men needed no longer to go to monastic centers for learning. Lay physicians reappeared in consequence. Meanwhile, Arabic influences revived the medical classics and a knowledge of these transcended the ordinary training of a monk. Gradually the Church itself discouraged priests from the practice of medicine, perhaps because this was no longer necessary under changed circumstances.

In due time lay physicians with university training organized professional guilds which, like other such bodies, tried to set standards and control practice. They admitted students to classes and also apprenticed them to older or master-physicians. University instruction was given entirely in terms of lectures and readings, and a man might take his medical degree without ever having seen a case. There was no such thing as clinical teaching, and no connection at first between

16 Selections quoted in MacKinney, 37, 38.

hospitals and medical schools. But the young doctor gained some experience during his apprenticeship, just as did a young carpenter or any other novice. And some governments began, late in the Middle Ages, to require that physicians be licensed by the state before they were allowed to practice.

Little emphasis was placed upon acquiring wealth in the profession. No doubt some doctors did become affluent but the Church discouraged such interests as sordid. Priests who practiced were supported by the Church and so rarely received money payments. Lay physicians were maintained by town authorities as municipal doctors and gave free care to the poor. Or they attached themselves to wealthy patrons. When the middle classes began to pay for medical service, the charges were controlled by the medical guild or "faculty." Hence medieval physicians were very conscious of their dignity. They felt that they were above vulgar competition and money-making. When modern conditions later forced doctors to compete with one another for fees— as once before in Roman days—there were difficult readjustments to make. Fears were expressed that the profession might become commercialized, like a business or a trade union. But even today, medical organizations are guided in part by surviving guild ideals.

The transfer to lay practice and the revival of Classical medicine can be first observed in southern Italy. Here Greco-Roman culture had never entirely disappeared and here also Arabic influences were first felt. A flourishing educational center appeared at Salerno, south of Naples, and during the tenth and eleventh centuries both clerical and lay physicians there acquired a wide reputation. Nearly 1200 students came regularly to the city for medical instruction and in this way the first medical faculty of Western Europe originated. Its members, some of whom had traveled in the East, were no longer satisfied with monastic writings. They read, instead, the works of Moslem physicians or Arabic translations from Greek classics. Eventually, Latin translations of Arabic translations of Hippocrates and Galen became available. Such works stimulated Salernitan physicians, in turn, to compose medical writings of their own. Once more, in this Italian center, texts began to be written on therapeutics, on surgery, and on hygiene.

An interesting feature of Salernitan writings is the information they provide about women physicians. One of them, the famous

Trotula, is supposed to have been a leader in the medical faculty there. Writings ascribed to her, especially those relating to pediatrics, were long popular. Certain authorities have questioned her existence, but it is hardly possible to deny that some women practiced medicine in the medieval period. It is difficult to distinguish, however, between those who practiced just because they were so inclined and those who secured some sort of professional training. In any case, this appearance of women physicians reminds one of their similar activity in Roman days. Later, when the universities developed, their faculties usually did not accept women for instruction. In some cases, as in Paris, action was taken to exclude women from all dignified, general practice; and their activities were limited to those of herbalists and midwives. Only in Italy, perhaps because the Roman tradition was strongest there, do a few women seem to have maintained university connections.

After 1250 the fame of Salerno became less than that of new universities such as Padua and Bologna in Italy, or Montpellier in France. The medical faculties in these new centers carried on in the tradition of Salerno, with the exception of one innovation which originated in the needs of forensic (legal) medicine. There had long been a belief that, in cases of suspected poisoning, an examination of the victim's body might prove whether or not murder had been committed. The law faculty at Bologna therefore suggested that dissections be made in such cases; and in 1315 one Mundinus, of the medical faculty there, responded by dissecting two bodies before his students.

The Church made no objection to this procedure on moral grounds, despite the fact that nothing had been heard of human dissections since the Alexandrian period several centuries before Christ. A precedent was thus established which was soon broadened to permit the dissection of executed criminals, and a way was opened for the study of human anatomy. (Salernitan anatomy, like that of Galen, had been limited to the structures of animals.) And, in time, human anatomy would become the very basis of modern medicine.

All this, however, lay far in the future. Human dissections remained rare for several centuries, and when made were not taken as seriously as were the Galenic writings. If structures described by Galen were not found, it was assumed that the dissector must be mistaken or the body abnormal! A century after Mundinus, anatomical drawings were still mere copies of those in Classical manuscripts, and a glance at such pictures will show how naive medieval notions of anatomy really were.

Lacking reliable knowledge of the basic sciences of anatomy and physiology, medicine continued to accept Galen's doctrine that all illness lay in the humors. Treatments therefore consisted of using vegetable drugs supposed to modify the humors, or of just ridding the body of these fluids by bleeding, sweating, and purging. Added to all this was some superficial surgery and a supplementary resort to religious healing.

As noted, medicine of this sort was reflected in Latin manuscripts written as guides for general practice. A good example is provided by the work of an English physician, John of Gaddesden (1280–1361), entitled *The Rose of England, the Practice of Medicine from the Head to the Feet.* Note, in the following excerpts, the references to Classical or Moslem authorities, to depletion procedures, to healing charms, and—last but not least—to claims about personal experience:[17]

PREFACE

Galen . . . says that it is impossible to come nearer to God by any other way than . . . by knowledge—therefore I have wished to write this book for the humble to read. Because since no book is written without reproach, as Galen says in the second book of his *de Crise,* so neither will this one be. But all the same, I implore those who see it . . . to read it through humbly, for nothing is set down here but what is proved by personal [bedside] experience, either of myself or others. . . .

ON HYDROPS [DROPSY]

Idropisis is a watery disease inflating the body. . . . Avicenna [an Arabic authority] says "Hydrops is an error of the combining energy of the whole body, following on a change of the digestive energy in the liver." The cure of hydrops is of two kinds, common and proper. . . . The first method is by diuretic medicines which provide a flow of urine such as spica, cassia and the like. The second method is to purge out the yellow fluid by means of sweating and discharge of the bowels. . . . The third method is for the patient to drink his own urine. . . . The fourth method is by means of an incision . . . below the umbilicus. . . . Avicenna says, "When the belly is full of water and the strength is well

17 Quoted in Logan Clendening, *Source Book of Medical History,* Paul B. Hoeber, Inc., New York, 1942, pp. 80 ff.

maintained, then make an incision and let out the water, but little by little and not all at once."

Again, when the gospel for Sunday is read in the mass, let the man hearing mass sign his tooth and his head with the sign of the Holy Cross and say a pater noster and an ave for the souls of the father and mother of St. Philip . . .; it will keep them from pain in the future and will cure that which may be present, so say trustworthy authorities.

The reference above to incisions recalls the matter of medieval surgery. Little distinction was made, during the period of monastic practice, between general medicine and surgery. Unfortunately, in later centuries, learned medical faculties came to disdain surgery as a trade involving merely manual skill; and they therefore relegated it to folk-practitioners. Routine surgery, like bleeding and tooth-pulling, were consequently taken over by the barber guilds. The red stripes on a barber's pole still recall this bleeding tradition.

Even serious operations, such as amputations or the removal of superficial tumors, were done by men trained only by apprenticeships. Procedures were crude and brutal. The use of ligatures was forgotten, and the hot iron was employed to stop hemorrhage or to destroy unhealthy tissues. To make matters worse, infection was expected and even welcomed by the operators. Wounds were not supposed to heal cleanly ("by first intention"), but rather "by second intention"—that is, with granulating surfaces and "laudable pus."

The latter phrase referred to a mistaken doctrine in Hippocrates which was carried over into modern times; namely, the view that pus in a wound was a good sign. For pus was supposed to result from a boiling process in the humors ("coction"), in which fluid impurities were brought to the surface and drained off. If pus did not appear, the surgeon feared that it was shut in and would damage the patient internally. Hence he welcomed the very signs of infection which today would be most dreaded. In a word, the acceptance of humoral theories was not only of little help but might also do positive harm. How anyone survived the shock and infection, following medieval or early modern operations, is something of a mystery.

A few able surgeons did appear, nevertheless, during the later Middle Ages. Such men attempted to use crude anesthetics and even employed aseptic, wine-soaked bandages. But they were handicapped by the general ignorance of anatomy and also by their uncertain professional status—midway between mere barber-surgeons on the one hand and learned "doctors" on the other.

Truly professional surgeons were notable in one way. Since they dealt with tangible structures in the body and were sure just what they were doing, they were inclined to be skeptical about the humoral theories of physicians. Hence some of the first protests against accepting Galenic authority were made by leading surgeons, who even questioned the doctrine of "laudable pus." Thus Henri de Mondeville, a famous French surgeon, declared in 1316 that "many more surgeons know how to cause suppuration than how to heal a wound." Do not follow Galen, he added, in allowing a wound to bleed, and "avoid the formation of pus, which is not a stage of healing, but a complication." Worried by constant citations of that Greco-Roman authority, de Mondeville protested sharply that "God did not exhaust all His creative power in making Galen."[18] It is unfortunate that such a critical attitude rarely appeared among medieval physicians.

Epidemics and Mental Illness

Neither internal medicine nor surgery exerted much control over disease conditions during the Middle Ages. Living conditions were more or less primitive and life-expectancy at birth was not half as high as it is at the present time. Despite a high birth rate, populations remained almost static—which is another way of saying that death rates were appalling. Children and young adults usually succumbed to infections. The minority of adults who lived long enough suffered from the usual chronic or degenerative disorders; but the incidence of these diseases cannot be estimated because they were rarely identified and there were in any case no statistics.

A few types of disease stand out in the record, nevertheless, because they were (1) dramatic, or (2) very widespread, or (3) of such a nature that something had to be done with the victims. In the first class belonged the epidemics, which terrorized people because of their sudden and unusual character. The most frightful epidemic disease was bubonic plague, which in 1348 wiped out whole villages and is estimated to have destroyed several million persons in that one year

[18] Quoted in F. H. Garrison, *The History of Medicine*, Philadelphia, 1929, p. 156.

("The Black Death"). Fortunately, "the plague" visited Europe only at long intervals. Most persistent and widespread of medieval diseases was a repulsive chronic infection called leprosy. So intense was the fear it aroused that even now this name (applied to what is probably a different disease) still frightens modern communities.

The disease type which most plainly demanded some provision for the victims was mental illness. Mild cases or the mentally deficient were tolerated at home, and every village had its "simple Simon." But the behavior of violent cases was objectionable or even dangerous, and such persons had to be "put away" somewhere. Special institutions were eventually set up for them in the larger towns. A well-known example of this was St. Mary's of Bethlehem in London, established about 1400. By common abbreviation the word Bethlehem became "Bedlam," and the latter term still symbolizes the confusion which prevailed in this place. Locks and chains were used there, though records also survive of those who were "restored to their senses."

Hippocrates had viewed mental illness as having natural causes, as when an excess of one humor (black bile) was said to produce "melancholia"—which is simply the Greek word for this fluid. As long as the Classical tradition prevailed, medieval writers maintained the Hippocratic view. But toward the end of the Middle Ages, such medical opinion was overshadowed by religious interpretations. Mental disorders had never been so easily explained by natural factors as had physical ills, and so there had always been a tendency to ascribe insane behavior to demons or evil spells.

Theologians finally elaborated supernatural explanations in terms of witchcraft; that is, the doctrines that (1) certain persons sold their souls to the Devil in return for magical powers, (2) these witches (women) or wizards (men) inflicted disease or other evils on their communities, (3) such persons could be suspected by their queer behavior, and (4) once recognized, they should be destroyed. The insane were certainly queer and so were often in danger of being called witches or wizards. Indeed, mere senility might make a person suspect, and many an "old hag" suffered a witch's death for no other reason. Persecution of this sort reached a climax during the religious excitement of the sixteenth century, when thousands of witches were tortured and burned in both Protestant and Catholic lands. Some, though not all, of these people were simply ill and should have been hospitalized rather than executed.

Preventive Medicine

Medieval peoples, like others, made efforts to prevent as well as to cure disease. In so far as illness was ascribed to religious factors, such as God's wrath or the Devil's designs, prayers or other devotional measures were employed to avoid it. Or, if astrological influences were feared, a man might consult horoscopes in time to escape a coming epidemic. When a famous surgeon was asked to explain "the Black Death," he blamed it on "the grand conjunction of the three superior planets, Saturn, Jupiter and Mars, in the sign of Aquarius. . . ."[19] Nowadays, we would blame it rather on a grand conjunction of rats and fleas, in the presence of certain bacteria.

Natural means for avoiding illness, however, were never entirely abandoned. Something of Classical hygiene survived in popular "health rules," which had a vogue with those who could afford to observe them. One of the most popular of Salernitan writings was a long poem giving a regimen for daily living, and including such sane advice as the famous couplet:

> Use three Physicians still; first Doctor Quiet,
> Next Doctor Merry-man, and Doctor Dyet.

Public hygiene was primarily a problem for the growing towns of the later period. With the breakdown of Roman sanitary engineering, water supplies became precarious and sewage systems largely nonexistent. Streets and houses are said to have been filthy. On the other hand, some authorities think the unsanitary condition of medieval communities has been exaggerated. It is known that towns maintained public baths of a crude sort and that some effort was made to keep the streets clean. Conditions were probably better, in some respects, than they were to be in the early modern centuries.

To the Middle Ages, moreover, is owed the revival of the belief in contagion which had been emphasized in ancient Jewish writings. While physicians sometimes overlooked this doctrine because it was ignored in Classical authorities, the people became convinced that such epidemic diseases as "the plague" passed from one person to an-

[19] Quoted in Victor Robinson, *The Story of Medicine*, New York, 1931, p. 231.

other. Biblical teachings encouraged this view. Hence a combination of folk medicine and religion encouraged early attempts to isolate the sick from the well, so as to protect the latter from contagion. The isolation of lepers was particularly severe—they were all forced to live apart in "lazar houses" or separate communities—and this practice may have contributed to the decline of the disease after 1400. A similar isolation of "lepers" is still required in the United States at the present time.

Evolution of Hospitals and Nursing

The general history of the Middle Ages, and that of medicine and hygiene in particular, provide a background for the evolution of hospitals and nursing during this epoch. Something has already been said about the appearance of Christian hospitals at the end of the Roman period. These provided care for all unfortunates—for orphans, the aged, and the sick. Most of those taken in were poor, but wayfarers of all sorts were also received.

During the early Middle Ages, disorderly conditions made it all the more necessary that hospitals should serve others beside the sick. A tenth-century English hostel was founded "to preserve travelers from being devoured by wolves and other voracious forest beasts." Some of these travelers were pilgrims visiting holy places (the English "Canterbury pilgrims" are well known in song and story); others were sick and sought healing shrines. That care extended to the ill and to the other travelers is well illustrated in the twelfth-century regulations of St. Mary's in Chichester, England. These read in part as follows:[20]

> If anyone in infirm health and destitute of friends should seek admission for a term, until he shall recover, let him be gladly received and assigned a bed. . . . In regard to the poor people who are received late at night, to go forth early in the morning, let the warden take care that their feet are washed, and, as far as possible, their necessities attended to.

In a word, the same building provided hospital beds and a night's lodging.

Early hospitals were founded and directed in various ways. The first were usually established by bishops in cathedral towns and remained under their control. Popes occasionally granted a hospital

[20] Quoted in R. M. Clay, *The Medieval Hospitals of England*, London, 1909, p. 5.

autonomy under papal supervision. As the cities grew, local guilds, town authorities, and private patrons also came into the picture by giving funds for such institutions. These gifts resulted from various motives—from pure benevolence, from a desire to do penance, or simply from a wish to rid the streets of distressing beggars. Endowments usually consisted of manors or farms, the products or income from which were given to the hospitals. But special gifts or local taxes were also made available in some cases.

Once endowed, a hospital had to be provided with an organization, buildings, and services. If under episcopal control, regulations were laid down or approved by the bishop. Administration was placed in the hands of a warden or rector who corresponded, roughly, to a modern superintendent. A large place also had its proctor or treasurer who managed the endowment and accounts. These officials were appointed by the bishop, or by private patrons with the bishop's consent.

In time, however, certain monastic orders also founded hospitals under their own direction. The early Benedictines, for example, provided infirmaries for their members and sometimes took in the local poor. More significant was the appearance, 1100–1400, of secular orders which made the care of the sick a primary duty. Among these groups were those established by St. Francis of Assisi, who was so appalled by the sufferings of lepers that he gave up all else to minister to them. The Franciscan friars who followed him lived in "the world," and in a simple, neighborly way did all they could to help the sick poor. A Franciscan order for women ("Poor Clares") devoted themselves to nursing those who were brought to them by the friars. Both these groups supported themselves by manual labor or by requesting alms.

One of the first orders which was originally planned to maintain hospitals was that of Santo Spirito or the Order of the Holy Ghost. This was founded by Guy de Montpellier about 1180, with the encouragement of Pope Innocent III. Governed by a Master-General at Rome and adopting the rule of St. Augustine, it established communities and hospitals all over Western Europe. By 1300 there were nearly two hundred of these; a century later there are said to have been as many as nine hundred. This was a male association. Similar in purpose was an order of sisters known as Oblates, founded in Florence in 1296. The latter served in the city hospitals, chiefly in Italy, and have been noted for their superior educational standards down to the present time.

The success of these "secular" orders was due in part to their relative freedom in the community. Unlike the stricter "regular" orders, whose rigid vows limited their opportunities to perform nursing services, friars or oblates took simple vows which permitted them to come and go as occasion required. During the later Middle Ages and in the Reformation period, the Church tended to require stricter rules of women's orders. This meant an emphasis on the contemplative ideal rather than on that of social service. As a result, the "Poor Clares" became an enclosed, austere order and their nursing services ceased. Since social need continued, however, other secular groups arose to meet it.

Among the latter were the famous Beguines of Flanders. Founded as early as 1184, these groups of women maintained a lay status, taking only simple vows to do welfare work in their communities. They could hold property, and leave the order and marry if they so desired. They gave their time to teaching, to making clothes, and to nursing in town hospitals. One is reminded here of the "Grey Ladies" or other women who volunteer to work in modern wards. In time, as the Beguines increased in numbers and wealth, they also built their own hospitals and administered them.

A sort of feminist note is to be observed in the desire of Beguines to be free of male control through bishops or monastic connections. One must recall that although Christianity recognized the spiritual equality of the sexes, lay women were actually more subordinated in medieval society than had been the women of the later Roman Empire. As Western civilization advanced, however, the status of women again began to improve. First signs of this can be seen in the independent spirit of these sisters, and in certain other phenomena like the rise of chivalry as a code for gentlemen. Both the secularism of the Beguines and their feminism—if one can call it that—anticipated modern tendencies.

The high regard of the church for nursing was made plain in the bestowal of sainthood on the leaders in this service. St. Francis is one example. Some of the most famous of the nursing saints were women, such as the beloved Elizabeth of Hungary and the learned Hildegarde of the Rhineland. The latter was a physician as well as nurse, and her

107

scientific knowledge was remarkable for the time. Such women were usually members of the nobility or leaders of secular communities, since these were the only spheres in which a woman was likely to possess the opportunity for extensive social activities.

A special type of nursing order appeared in the military brotherhoods which arose out of the Crusades and other wars. Hostels for pilgrims going to Jerusalem had been established in Palestine during the early Middle Ages. With the capture of Jerusalem by crusaders about 1100, Christian soldiers and their retainers needed hospital facilities there. Groups of knights thereupon sought to provide such institutions, and out of this movement grew the famous Knights Hospitallers of St. John of Jerusalem. The crusading spirit lent some luster to this organization and it acquired lands and wealth throughout the Mediterranean world. Like other orders, it was independent of diocesan authorities and was governed by its Grand Master along military lines. Primary attention was given to military hospitals. Each of these was under a "Commander," and was served by three classes of members—priests, knights, and "serving brothers." The latter probably did the real nursing. Because of their wealth, the order's chief hospitals at Jerusalem, Rhodes, and Malta were better equipped than any others of the period, and they probably influenced all the larger hospitals of the later Middle Ages.

The Hospitallers may have learned something of planning and administration from the hospitals of the Byzantine Empire and also from those of Moslem lands in the Near East. The former were usually superior to those of Latin Europe until the time of the Crusades. At Alexandria, for example, a male order of nurses long served in the hospitals before any such groups were well organized in the West. When the Moslems took over the greater part of the Eastern Empire and absorbed Greek medicine, they also established hospitals more elaborate than those existing in the Latin world. They profited from the example of the old hospitals of India when they established their first institutions in Bagdad, Cairo, and other centers. These were served by both men and women as nurses. (Mohammedanism, like Christianity and Judaism, taught charity towards the poor.) How far the Moslem institutions provided medical as well as custodial care, however, is not clear.

The Knights Hospitallers were finally expelled from Palestine along with other Christians about 1300. Subsequently they maintained themselves in Rhodes until 1522, and held Malta until Napoleon drove them out in 1798. Their substantial hospital buildings can still be seen on both islands. Maintaining a semi-military tradition, the Hospitallers have survived in Europe as units supplying ambulance and other medical services during recent wars. But their original functions have been largely taken over and expanded during the last century by the International Red Cross.

Other military orders which originated in Palestine and later spread back to Europe, were the Knights Templars and the Teutonic Knights. With them, however, emphasis was placed upon military rather than upon nursing services. Both the Hospitallers and the Teutonic Knights formed women's orders which performed hospital work; but as often happened, these groups seem to have been subordinated to the men's communities.

Development of Medical Care in Hospitals

Estimates of the number of hospitals built in medieval Europe are necessarily inexact but give some idea of the scale of the movement involved. It is stated, for example, that between 1207 and 1577, over one hundred and fifty were set up in Germany alone. Unfortunately, such figures give no measure of size. Large numbers of village "homes" contained only about a dozen beds. Town hospitals, on the other hand, attained a considerable scale by the fourteenth century. St. Leonard's in York, for example, provided in 1370 some two hundred and twenty-five beds. Probably the largest of medieval hospitals was Santo Spirito in Rome, which by 1500 possessed a main hall containing nearly one thousand beds. So large an institution also included several distinct wards, providing respectively for men, for women, and for convalescents.

With advances in the arts and some increase in wealth, the buildings and equipment of hospitals improved during the later Middle Ages. The larger institutions were housed in beautiful Gothic structures, similar in architectural form to the churches of the period. Indeed, the appearance of a main hall or ward would have suggested an ecclesiastical interior to a modern observer. (When churches were commandeered during recent wars to serve as emergency hospitals, the resulting arrangements looked more like early hospitals than the doctors realized.) Straw pallets were replaced by wooden beds, and curtains or partitions supplied some privacy. Linen and woolen supplies became more ample, and a large place would have its own farms to provide food and its own wind or water mills to prepare "corn" (wheat) for the patients. Although the buildings were still cold and dark by modern standards, they were a great improvement over the bare and humble dwellings of the "dark ages."

The actual care of hospital patients during the early Middle Ages was largely custodial in nature. It was provided, as noted, partly by monks or nuns and partly by servants. Just where the work of "the religious" stopped and that of servants began is difficult to say. The point is of some interest, since one of the difficulties in setting up the modern nursing profession was to disentangle it from a servant tradition. Romans had assigned nursing to servants or slaves. Hence, when early Christian gentlewomen served in hospitals, it was viewed as a special virtue that they carried food and did "all those other things which are reckoned the work of slaves or handmaidens."[21] No doubt these women and the later "religious" did much, though not all, of the more personal nursing. But routine work, such as cleaning floors, was assigned to servants in the larger institutions.

The environment in which this personnel labored was, during the earlier centuries, an almost entirely religious one. Although simple medical attention was provided, prayers and services were the chief feature of the daily routine. The strictest observances were expected of the nursing brothers or sisters in view of their religious vows. But even the patients were expected to say their prayers by day and by night. A brother or sister woke them for this purpose. In addition to religious purposes, such services may have been intended to maintain discipline and morale. Patients were at times disorderly, and some might just wander out when so inclined. Wardens, in order to deal with such problems, were usually authorized to impose fasts or floggings or to expel as a last resort.

During the later medieval period, the revival of a lay medical profession brought physicians into the hospitals. The most reputable of these men were those who had attended universities, knew Latin translations of Greek and Arabic medical writings, and had received

[21] Quoted in Lucy R. Seymer, *A General History of Nursing,* New York, 1939, p. 30.

the degree of doctor of medicine—just as others had become doctors of law or of philosophy. Hospital authorities, anxious to provide what seemed the best medicine to their patients, welcomed these learned doctors into their halls. The latter, when they followed a patient into the hospital or were called in to see one, viewed this as a charitable service. But if a large institution asked a physician to attend many patients regularly, they might pay him a retainer fee.

In any case, a connection was thus established between physicians and hospitals which would eventually prove significant for science as well as for charity. In the Roman hospital already mentioned (Santo Spirito), more than one hundred physicians and surgeons are said to have been in attendance. And by the fourteenth and fifteenth centuries, this and other large institutions were beginning to develop modern forms of professional service. Thus, at Santa Maria Nuova in Florence, three young, resident doctors reported daily on each patient to six visiting physicians. The same hospital maintained a dispensary for out-patients in which drugs were provided free to the poor. It is even claimed that medical students occasionally observed treatments in the hospitals, though such use of the wards for clinical training was certainly rare for several centuries thereafter.

Hospital Administration and Practices

Up to this point, the account given of medieval hospitals and nursing orders has necessarily been general in nature. A more specific description of a single hospital may serve, in conclusion, to make the whole picture more real. One can take for this purpose the famous Hôtel-Dieu of Paris, for which unusually complete records survive.

Built near the Cathedral of Notre Dame, the Hôtel-Dieu already possessed five wards and a complicated organization during the thirteenth century. It was ruled by a prior (warden) under episcopal authority, with a prioress in charge of the sisters who did most of the actual nursing. Both brothers and sisters belonged to strict, regular orders following the rule of St. Augustine. Their activities may be classified as (1) exterior work, (2) hospital administration, (3) care of the sick, and (4) religious services. Under the first heading came the management of farms which were a part of the endowment. This work was supervised by the brothers.

Hospital administration involved the admission, discharge, and

111

burial of patients, provision of food and drink, and the care of bedding and clothing. Certain brothers were in charge of corresponding departments. Making provision in these respects for several hundred patients—without "modern conveniences" and with few labor-saving devices—was no small matter. The younger sisters or novices, for example, did all the washing nearby on the banks of the Seine.

The patients, admitted by a sister at the gate, were directed to the appropriate hall and here distributed two or more to a bed. This was later viewed as infamous overcrowding, but it is to be remembered that similar arrangements were then customary in families. (The modern sense of privacy, along with other luxuries, could be cultivated only when living standards rose after 1500. Indeed, some Latin peoples have never developed it to the degree now common in English-speaking lands.) Yet there were always some patients who did have beds to themselves.

Some nursing in the general wards was done by brothers but all that in the women's ward was in the hands of sisters. The latter went through three stages of training, and their labor and devotion were great indeed. Besides tending the kitchens, washing, and so on, they admitted and discharged patients and buried the dead. Servants seem to have been available only for the most humble work, such as cleaning the floors.

The sisters rose at five, and went to chapel while the Prioress made her first tour of inspection. At six they went to their various labors, those in the wards putting out the lights and tending the sick. While beds were made, the patients rose if possible or were placed temporarily on other couches. (The modern art of giving baths and changing linen without moving the patient had not yet evolved.) The sisters served two meals per day in the wards, and went out on relays to secure the same number for themselves. The regulations directed that patients should receive anything wholesome which they desired to eat but it is hard to believe that this was the actual practice.

Similar duties occupied the sisters during the afternoon. At seven they retired to their dormitory, while "watchers" were left in the halls and the prioress made one last night round guided by a torch. The records speak realistically of the difficulty which the sisters experienced in enjoying the evening meal, after hours spent amid unpleasant odors and trying scenes. They seem to have had little if any time for recreation, and there is no indication that they received any medical instruction other than that involved in practical experience.

At the Hôtel-Dieu, as elsewhere, religious rites were an essential part of hospital procedure. Services were conducted for both patients and staff, and individuals were offered consolation and the sacraments. Funeral services were held, and prayers said for patrons and benefactors.

It would be a strange experience if one could be transported back to such a busy, medieval hospital, and so to actually observe these activities which we now know only through musty documents. Much would seem unfamiliar, perhaps even disturbing. The lack of privacy, of sanitary standards, and of scientific procedures would be woefully apparent. Yet a discerning eye would also observe a fine devotion and —in the total setting—the prototype of our present-day institutions.

Chapter VI

Renaissance and Reformation:

New Methods Mould a New Science

It is no more possible to say just when the Middle Ages ended than it is to decide just when they began. Much that was medieval survived into the early modern centuries. American colonists were still using Gothic architecture, for example, as late as 1700—as anyone who looks at the oldest colonial buildings can see. Medieval influences survive, for that matter, at the present time. All one can say is that great changes began in European life as early as 1250, that these were accelerated after 1450, and that by about 1750 so-called modern characteristics had become dominant in western Europe.

These dates are only approximate ones, because changes came at different times in different countries, and also occurred at various intervals according to the phase of culture concerned. Thus serfdom, a feudal form of labor, was abolished in England before 1600, in France in 1790, but in Russia not until 1860. Again, the science of physics was modern in character by 1650, but medicine was still medieval in some ways a century later. Nevertheless, there were periods when change was relatively rapid and spread from one land to another in such a way as to give a new tone to many phases of life. The most striking of these periods was that usually called the Renaissance, which began in Italy about 1450 and whose spirit permeated western Europe during the ensuing century. It is usually viewed as the chief period of transition from medieval to modern times.

The influences which brought about the Renaissance, whether of an economic, scientific, or religious character, were complex and varied. All acted simultaneously, and one separates them in retrospect only as a convenience for historical analysis. Thus, the confiscation of church properties by Henry VIII of England involved political, economic, and religious factors all operating at the same time. This action, incidentally, involved the hospitals and naturally affected the doctors and nurses therein. One has here, therefore, an illustration of the fact that neither medical science nor medical care could escape the transformations which ushered in the modern age.

Extension of Commerce

Economic developments were certainly a major factor in bringing about the Renaissance. After the wars between Moslems and Christians ceased, trade between them increased. Oriental goods from as far as India and China were brought to Alexandria and other eastern Mediterranean ports, were thence carried by Italian merchants to Genoa or Venice, and were then passed on to the towns of northern Europe. Italians were the middlemen in these exchanges and they waxed wealthy in the process. Businessmen became the dominant class in their cities and were led by merchant-princes like the Medici of Florence. As late as Shakespeare's day (1600), it was the "Merchant of Venice" who impressed Englishmen as the dynamic type of business leader.

Life on rural manors, in contrast, had been simple and did not make for change. Serfs were held to the soil, ignorant and isolated. The nobles wished only to fight or to follow the easygoing ways of a landed aristocracy. They despised townspeople as sordid money-makers and termed them "commoners" or "bourgeoisie." Until very recently, indeed, English aristocrats looked down on those who "went into trade" (business), and there is still social prestige in the life of a "country gentleman." Nothing new was likely to come out of a static society of this sort.

Just the opposite was true of the towns. Here the businessmen and workers were in close contact with one another and exchanged ideas as well as goods. Competition forced them to be aggressive and to seek new ways of doing things. Modern business forms and methods, for example, were first introduced by Italian merchants. Among these were the use of Arabic numerals, of bookkeeping, and of the insurance principle of sharing losses among a large number of people. The Italians also revived the use of money, which had seemed unnecessary on feudal manors but was so useful in trade. The towns used money to employ soldiers and fleets and so made themselves independent of the nobility.

The use of gold and silver coins, moreover, undermined the power of aristocrats even on their own estates. Noblemen also desired foreign goods that only money could buy; to secure funds they gradually freed their serfs from forced labor and rented land to them for cash payments. A serf's labor could only bring in food, but rent payments could be used by the lord for any purpose. In this way, many serfs finally became free men independent of feudal control.

Development of the Fine Arts

Meanwhile, in the towns, the wealth of merchant princes afforded them leisure and an opportunity to cultivate the arts. Hitherto, only Church institutions had been able to do this and these had naturally employed artists primarily for religious ends. Medieval musicians and architects devoted themselves, respectively, to church music and to church buildings. Painting had been limited almost entirely to religious subjects such as one can see in the "Italian primitives" in any large museum. But merchants were naturally worldly. They enjoyed the comforts of this world and their interests tended to center in it. They desired palaces rather than cathedrals, and painters in their employ depicted contemporary life rather than idealized themes from the Christian tradition.

In Italian Renaissance painting, it is true, religious subjects still predominated. Here the popes and other church authorities continued to be among the chief patrons of art. But it is plain that artists were becoming interested in a faithful reproduction of natural objects. They portrayed real people with increasing skill in perspective and color, until such masterpieces were attained as Leonardo da Vinci's "Last Supper." The same trend was carried further among Flemish and Dutch masters, who frankly abandoned religious themes altogether and devoted themselves to portraits of merchants or princes and even to scenes from everyday life. One of the activities which interested Dutch artists was the drama of human dissection, as already

117

practiced in their medical schools. Hence they left excellent portrayals of this stage of medical research, as in Rembrandt's classic "Lesson in Anatomy." More than this, certain artists were of direct service to medicine through their masterly illustrations of the anatomic texts of the period. They knew anatomy well, since they studied it to perfect their portrayal of human bodies. This was a great age in medical art.

Renaissance painting was "realistic" in that it sought to reproduce natural objects as these actually appeared. This was in contrast to the conventionalized figures of earlier "primitives," which now seem crude because most people since the Renaissance have desired realistic effects. For the same reason, most of us today are confused by the reappearance of abstract, unrealistic painting in so-called modernistic forms. But from the point of view of general history, the striking thing about Renaissance painting is its human quality, as contrasted with the other-worldly, religious emphasis of medieval creations. One can see, in this one art, an expression of that secular, "humanistic" outlook which gradually permeated all aspects of Renaissance life.

Development of the Practical Arts

While expressions of secular tendencies were to be found in the fine arts, the forces actually producing these trends were more closely associated with the practical arts. It was noted in the preceding chapter that, throughout the later Middle Ages, master-workmen in the guilds were slowly improving their products. Growing skill in glass-making and in metal-working has been mentioned. Technical progress was especially noticeable in the maritime arts. Merchants wished to improve shipbuilding and sailing methods and, as usual, necessity was the mother of invention. They learned to sail close to the wind rather than merely before it, and so had less need of oars. (Anyone who can "tack" in a sailboat knows what this means.) The mariners' compass, long known in the East, was brought to Europe after the Crusades and proved a great help to navigation when seamen were out of sight of land or stars.

Another invention brought from China was gunpowder, which the Europeans employed in firearms. Eventually such weapons changed the methods of war, for armored knights on horseback were no match for this sort of artillery. Gunpowder, like money, would do much to destroy feudalism.

These technologic improvements were, to be sure, sometimes scorned by learned scholars who did not deign to work with their hands. Pure science was still largely, in 1450, a matter of "book-learning." But the scholastic barrier between science and technology began to break down. When the Venetians set up an arsenal to study artillery and the motion of cannon balls toward a target, they found Arabic numerals useful in these technical observations. Later their debt to science was repaid, when Galileo used their work to aid him in developing the pure mathematics of moving bodies (dynamics). So science and technology began to be mutually useful as early as 1600, and their interaction speeded up social change of many kinds.

Another illustration of the interdependence of practical arts and science—indeed of practical art and all intellectual activity—is to be seen in the greatest of Renaissance inventions. This was the printing press, with which letters could be stamped on paper by movable type. This also had been known long before in China and the idea may have come in with the Oriental trade. The first complete European book to be printed in this way was the famous Gutenberg Bible (1454), a copy of which may be seen in the Library of Congress. Only a limited number of works were printed before 1500. Rare examples of these early printings are known as "incunabula" (from Latin for "in the cradle"; that is, the beginnings), and are now among the most highly-prized books in existence. After 1500 manuscripts were rapidly superseded by printed volumes. So many copies could be made quickly that books became much cheaper and more common than ever before.

The significance of this change can hardly be exaggerated. Whereas manuscripts had always been very rare and only the wealthy or members of religious orders could secure them, all educated men could now read the printed words. New ideas, already in circulation in certain centers, could spread rapidly all over Europe. Such a movement as the Reformation could hardly have aroused northern Europe as it did, had it not been for the ease with which Luther's writings circulated throughout the whole region. And this was true of any new viewpoint. Eventually, nearly every aspect of life was changed in consequence. Thus scientists, long isolated from one another save by occasional correspondence, were able to read one another's books and exchange ideas promptly. In time, periodicals appeared for the even more rapid exchange of thought. Without printing, the later scientific societies and their publications would have been quite impossible. Thus did a single device promote a revolution in science and in all other fields of learning.

The influence of printing is also to be seen in the revival of classical art and science in the Renaissance period. It has been noted that, in the later Middle Ages, scholars prepared Latin translations from Arabic translations of the original Greek and Roman manuscripts. In time, translations directly from the Greek began to be made. In this way the Italians recovered their original heritage without having to take it second-hand from the Moslems. Constantinople, where Greco-Roman culture survived, became a center for their labors. When this last remnant of the Roman Empire finally fell to the Turks about 1450, Greek scholars fled to Italy and further stimulated these interests. Ancient philosophers like Plato and Aristotle, Greek and Roman physicians like Galen and Celsus, and classical writers in general were once more read as they had been in their own days. Then printing spread this classical lore from Italy all over Europe during the 1500's. An edition of the forgotten medical encyclopedia of Celsus's, for example, was published at Florence in 1478; and knowledge of this and of other classical medical works became widespread during ensuing decades.

The eagerness with which scholars, merchants, and many churchmen welcomed revived classical writings, is itself evidence of their changing viewpoint. Greeks and Romans had centered their interests in human, worldly affairs, and the men of the Renaissance found that they once more shared this outlook. A love for "pagan" literature would have been deemed dangerous, if not heretical, in an earlier day when Greek learning had been followed only for the purpose of fitting it into Christian theology. Now this worldly culture was once more pursued for its own sake. Here again the Renaissance leaders displayed primarily human rather than theological enthusiasms, and they have been known ever since as "humanists."

The Europeans of 1500 were "catching up" with the secular culture which had always survived in Moslem and Byzantine lands. But they did more than catch up. For in the Roman and Greek authors they found an originality, an independence which struck a responsive cord. With new wealth and new vistas, the Italians felt able to take up where classical art and science had "left off." Gone was the long preoccupation with other-worldly, religious concerns. These men meant to live in this world and to make the most of it. Did they not have tools and weapons with which even the Romans had been unfamiliar? They would use classical art and science, to be sure, but not merely to imitate it. They would improve upon it.

Such enthusiasms had an intoxicating effect upon the artists and thinkers of the day. Their ideal became the perfection of human personality and they wished no bonds on the individual's search for such perfection. This meant extreme freedom in thought and action, especially for the genius in self-expression. In no era since the best days of Athens, were so many brilliant and versatile individuals produced as appeared in Italy between 1450 and 1600. Leonardo da Vinci, perhaps the outstanding genius of all time in both art and science, well illustrates the type. On the other hand, this extreme freedom also led to license and to an abandonment of the moral standards of the medieval Church. One gathers, in reading the autobiography of such an artist as Benvenuto Cellini, that he viewed the world solely in terms of the gratification of his own desires.

This state of mind also brought with it a sense of emancipation from the immediate past. There was a strong desire to abandon everything medieval. The word "Gothic" (in architecture) was then invented as meaning the crude and primitive—a term of reproach. Italian architects forsook the pointed arches and buttressed walls of Gothic forms, and went back to Roman ruins for inspiration. Dignified, symmetrical buildings with round, Roman arches came into vogue. But they did not merely imitate imperial temples and baths. Rather they adapted classical ideas to their own needs. Florentine palaces showed classical details but were new in form. The flat dome of the Pantheon in Rome was superseded by the great, soaring dome of St. Peter's Cathedral—a type which later became popular in American capitols. Eventually, Italian Renaissance architecture developed elaborate details and influenced similar forms in Spain and Northern Europe in the so-called baroque styles of the seventeenth century. The old buildings of Mexico express the Spanish form of this movement; the Georgian or "Colonial" structures in the United States represent the English version.

Development of Nationalism and Exploration

While popes and merchant-princes were the chief supporters of art in Italy, kings became the most wealthy patrons in Spain, France, and England. This reflected a significant difference in political trends; for although Italy remained a land divided between many city-states, unified kingdoms were developing in the other countries named. This unity was largely achieved through the monarchs, who were supported by towns in gradually overthrowing feudal lords and in adding many small principalities to the royal domains.

As the national territory expanded, other changes occurred. Gradually the language and customs of the capital were extended throughout the whole kingdom. Thus, the language now called French was once only the dialect spoken around Paris. As the people in different provinces came to speak this, and to adopt also the manners and customs of Paris, they began to feel that they were all Frenchmen and should be true to France as a whole. Although this process was never entirely completed—there are still several different languages spoken in France and also within other European countries—the trend was clear. The process was encouraged by growing pride in a national language and culture. Literary men began to work in their own tongue instead of simply in Latin, as when Dante wrote in Italian and Chaucer in English, and this established a standardized, national speech. Eventually, these "modern languages" would replace Latin even in learned publications.

Loyalty to the nation, or patriotism, was also aroused by wars against other peoples. Thus St. Joan of Arc stirred the French people in her heroic campaigns against English invaders. And the several Spanish principalities were welded together in their common crusades against the Moors. When the last Moslem territory was finally conquered by Isabella of Castile and by Ferdinand of Aragon in 1492, these two monarchs married and so united the whole Spanish peninsula except for Portugal. By the same time, Henry VII of England and Charles VIII of France each ruled over fairly well united peoples and territories.

These monarchs acquired greater power than even the city-states of Italy could command. Naturally they were ambitious to surpass the latter in wealth as well, and they looked with jealous eyes on Italian trade with the Orient. So arose the desire to find new routes to the East, by which the western nation-states could compete with the Italians. Here a reviving knowledge of Greek geography came to their aid, by suggesting that the world was round and that the East could therefore be reached by sailing west around the globe. Of great aid also were the improved methods of sailing and navigation already noted. Italians were still the best sea-captains; and everyone knows how Ferdinand and Isabella employed one of them, Columbus, to make his great voyage in 1492. As a result he found, not the East Indies, but a whole new world.

The French and English kings also sent Italian explorers to America; but the Spaniards secured a head start in founding colonies there and in drawing wealth from this growing Empire. Meanwhile, the Portuguese found their way to the East Indies by sailing around Africa; and in this way they as well as other Atlantic seaboard nations took the Oriental trade away from the Italians. New wealth began pouring into Spain and Portugal, and somewhat later into France, England, and Holland; and this wealth promised much for subsequent cultural progress in those nations.

While powerful nation-states were thus forming in Western Europe, Central Europe remained disunited. Germany, as will be seen, was torn by religious struggles, and Italy was divided by the jealousies of city-states. Also located in Italy were the popes, who had no desire to come under the control of any national state. Their religious authority reached through the Church into every Catholic country and was independent of secular governments. It was this very fact, however, which aroused anti-clerical feeling among the more aggressive monarchs, who saw in the international Church an obstacle to the exercise of complete power within their own borders.

Religious Revolt and Reformation

Nationalism was not the only development which tended to disturb the position of the Church. Humanistic trends produced a ferment *within* the Church, at the same time that monarchs threatened it from *without*. When Italian leaders abandoned the outlook of medieval Christianity, they lost interest in maintaining that tradition. Not only did artists and scientists live as they chose but they also desired freedom to think as they saw fit. Critical of the past and optimistic about the future, some of them questioned both the doctrine and practices of orthodox religion. They ridiculed the Church in private though they rarely opposed it openly. This undermining of traditional beliefs and morals even affected some of the leading clergy. The latter became tolerant of private beliefs, and were themselves patrons of the arts and good living in the most cultivated Renaissance manner. A spirit of "live and let live" developed in which the arts and sciences flourished, and Italy seemed to be adjusting religious tradition to the new outlook in an urbane and peaceful manner.

Far different was the outcome in northern lands. Here, when scholars questioned the doctrine or practice of the Church, other forces came into play which were absent in the south. The wealth and sophistication of the Church in Italy seemed to poorer Germans and Englishmen a sign of worldliness. They resented, moreover, the fact that some of this wealth was taken from their own countries to Rome, through the taxing powers and other procedures of the Church. This attitude was especially true of the middle classes, who as business men lived a sober life and wanted to keep their money at home. But similar resentment was displayed by kings and princes, who not only wanted to keep money at home but wished also to add to their funds by taxing or seizing Church properties within their own borders. Monarchs further disliked the fact that ecclesiastical authorities maintained courts and exercised other powers within their kingdoms, and so prevented civil governments from securing complete control of the people. Increasing friction therefore developed between the old authority of the Church and the new power of the State.

So it was that when critics of the Church arose in Germany, they received support from both townspeople and princes. And this led eventually to open revolt. The grounds of criticism were at first partly the same as were privately expressed in Italy. Humanist scholars, like Erasmus in Holland, deplored the wealth and worldliness of some of the clergy. But it was soon noticeable that a strong sense of moral protest was developing in Germany. The Renaissance interest in Classical culture led certain German scholars to reexamine the original Christian scriptures (the Bible), and they maintained that all beliefs and practices not found by them in these scriptures should be abandoned. The Church, these reformers held, should repudiate the

Middle Ages—even as artists had done—and return to the purity and simplicity of apostolic days.

This was an historical appeal back to the authority of the Bible, as against the traditional authority of the papacy and of the Church Councils. It led to much searching of the Old and New Testaments, in the course of which various views appeared as to what the doctrines, government, and services of the Church should be. Sooner or later, under these circumstances, sharp differences of opinion were bound to appear. The major controversy was precipitated by Martin Luther, a German monk who in 1517 publicly protested against the purchase of "indulgences" for certain sins. Neither the Pope nor the Emperor[22] succeeded in suppressing him, since German princes promptly took him under their protection. The controversy was carried far and wide by printed pamphlets and soon broadened to include all aspects of Christianity. Luther's followers became known as Lutherans and also as Protestants—because they "protested" against papal authority. They soon declared the independence of their congregations from the pope and the right of each state—which meant each prince—to choose between the new Church and the old.

Protestant princes in Germany, following this view, promptly revealed their nationalistic motives. They made themselves the heads of the Lutheran Church in their respective territories, required all their subjects to accept it, seized church lands and buildings, and suppressed convents and monasteries. Luther translated the Bible so that all could read the scriptures in their own tongue and he also advocated some modifications of Catholic doctrine and ritual. Soon the greater part of northern Germany had adopted his standard.

Meanwhile, the success of Lutheranism encouraged other revolts from Catholic authority. In Switzerland, John Calvin developed another version of Protestanism which emphasized a strict and pious— though not celibate—life for all believers. Services were made simple and severe. This system appealed particularly to the sober business classes of northern Europe, and it spread into France, Holland, and the British Isles. In these lands it was known, respectively, as the Huguenot, the Reformed, and the Presbyterian movement.

Both the Lutheran and Calvinistic groups established dignified

[22] Of the shadowy "Holy Roman Empire," which had come down from Charlemagne's time.

churches, each under the control of the State and as intolerant of opposition as was Catholicism. Much the same thing may be said of the Church of England, the immediate cause of whose organization was the conflict between Henry VIII and the pope over the former's demand for a divorce. Actually, however, the Church of England was formed as a result of certain forces making for Protestantism in general. Henry seized church properties just as had the German princes, and closed hospitals as well as monasteries. Meanwhile, Lutherans, Calvinists, and Anglicans could not agree among themselves. This revealed an organizational weakness in Protestantism; namely, the fact that if the Bible were the chief source of authority, there might be almost as many interpretations thereof as there were readers. And who was to decide between them?

Each of these Protestant churches answered this question by setting up its own authority, as in the Augsburg Confession of the Lutherans or the Thirty-nine Articles of the Church of England. But this did not satisfy all the people in their respective countries. Many found other meanings in the scriptures and formed groups like the Baptists, who agreed neither with Catholicism nor with conservative State Protestantism. Some were poor folk, who resented the aristocratic control of State churches and who fused religious questions with strivings for social betterment. They demanded a complete separation of Church and State, so that no civil power could be used against any faith or doctrine. Since they were persecuted by the State churches, they called for religious freedom. These men, as individuals, felt that they were in direct communion with God, and this made a church organization or clergymen seem largely unnecessary to them. Nor did they desire the aid of ritual or ceremonies in such a communion. The English Friends (Quakers) were an example of this type of Protestantism.

The more ignorant of these lowly folk were apt to interpret the Bible in ways that seemed strange and bizarre to the educated classes. All sorts of new movements appeared, some wild and undisciplined, and these carried their dislike of everything Catholic to extremes. Statues of saints were smashed, stained-glass windows were demolished, and radical individualism of all kinds threatened religious chaos. The more extreme wing of Protestantism seemed in danger of disintegration.

While all this was going on, efforts to reconcile Catholicism and Protestantism failed. The Catholic Church, in an effort to meet some of the criticisms of reformers and also to organize its opposition to Protestantism, instituted changes known as the Counter Reformation. From 1545 to 1563, a great Council was held at Trent in northern Italy, which reformed serious abuses, adopted a simple, popular prayer book, and instilled a more rigorous discipline which was destined to affect nursing orders as well as other groups.

Europe then drifted into a tragic struggle between Catholic and Protestant countries. The latter were chiefly in northern Europe, where middle-class interests and national sentiment were strongest. There is no need to follow here the long story of these struggles, in which selfish or national ambitions became inextricably confused with religious sentiments. Suffice it to say that while much was gained for individual rights and church reform in these conflicts, there is also no question that many of the results were unfortunate. The wars increased bitterness and bigotry on both sides, which even now has not entirely disappeared. A terrible example of this is to be seen in the witchcraft persecutions, which revealed a reversion to a super- stitious theology in all lands. The services of hospitals and other charities suffered from their temporary suppression. And as Europe was now permanently divided along religious as well as along national- istic lines, the medieval ideal of a united, Western Christendom became only a memory.

Science Moves Forward

If one concentrated entirely on the religious history of the Ren- aissance period, it might lead to the impression that all men became preoccupied with religious conflicts. Yet this was far from the case. Wherever one faith or another was entirely dominant, there was little internal discord. Thus in Italy, where Protestantism took little hold, the arts and sciences continued to flourish. Conversely, in Holland and in England, where Catholicism almost disappeared, Renaissance culture spread rapidly from Italy. Only in lands which were bitterly divided on religious grounds, notably in Germany, did civil war seri- ously retard the advance of civilization.

It is well, therefore, to return to the major theme of cultural change in the Renaissance era. The whole Reformation struggle was, in a sense, the religious phase of this process. The most significant aspect of the Renaissance which has not yet been considered is that of science. This type of human activity was not directly involved in the religious quarrels, for—as was also true of art—it could be and was cultivated alike by Catholics, by Protestants, and by Jews. It was confined to no particular nationality or creed.

Science, as well as art, profited from the revival of Classical culture without being subservient to it. Renaissance scholars learned much from the new publications of Greek physics, geography, and medicine; but at the same time displayed a critical attitude towards this learning and an inclination to improve upon it. Mathematicians, using Arabic arithmetic and algebra, were able to trace more exactly the movements of the sun, moon and planets. Most of the Greek and practically all medieval thinkers had held that these heavenly bodies circled about the earth—as anyone could see for himself! This view made man's world the center of the universe. But during the sixteenth century Copernicus, an Italian-trained, Polish astronomer, declared that the earth and planets moved about the sun. If so, the earth was not the center of creation after all. What is more, he demonstrated that their movements could be better measured and explained from this point of view.

As did all good scientific ideas, the Copernican theory suggested more questions and further research. What kept the earth from falling into the sun? How fast did it move? What were the "laws" of moving bodies in general, on earth as well as in the heavens? An Italian with medical training, the famous Galileo, devoted himself to these questions and especially to the study of falling objects. It was difficult to observe things which just happened to fall—he was usually not there at the time. He therefore climbed the Leaning Tower of Pisa and proved that light objects fell as rapidly as heavy ones. This was startling, because Aristotle had said—and "common sense" still suggests —that heavy bodies drop more rapidly. Galileo also rolled balls down measured inclines to show how much faster they went the longer they were in motion, and so discovered the "law of acceleration."

In all this research the Italian physicist was constantly experimenting and measuring. Each of these processes extended the range of observation in general. Experimentation revealed hitherto unobserved phenomena—things a passive onlooker would never see. Measurement

128

enabled one to note accurately what was otherwise only a vague observation. Galileo did not invent these methods; they had been used by a few Classical scientists many centuries before. Again, toward the end of the Middle Ages, mathematicians had become interested in measuring the motion of physical bodies and Galileo's studies emerged from this background. Experimentation and measurement, moreover, were "in the air" by his time, because of the work of alchemists and that of skilled artisans—as in the Venetian arsenal where Galileo made some of his studies.

Galileo, nevertheless, employed these methods more systematically and effectively than anyone had done before his time. Knowing the theories of the mathematicians, he was not too proud to combine these with the practical knowledge possessed by mechanics and artillerymen; and as a result he really demonstrated what others had speculated about. Since his day, it has been taken for granted that any science will employ experiment and measurement as far as is possible; and some have even held that, without these methods, no field can be truly scientific in nature.

One other procedure, unknown to either Greek or medieval thinkers, was necessary to set science on the track of its modern achievements. This procedure was the use of devices to improve observation in a third way; namely, through instruments to aid the senses. Here again, practical artisans came to the aid of pure research. In Holland the lens-grinders, who had been making spectacles for more than two centuries, found that a combination of lenses would magnify objects. Hearing of this, Galileo put lenses in a tube and made one of the first telescopes. Looking through this at the sky, he saw what human eyes had never seen before—mountain craters on the moon, and great rings of light sweeping around Saturn. Anyone who looks at the heavens for the first time through a modern telescope can sense the thrill he experienced.

Armed with these three aids to observation—experimentation, measurement, and instruments to improve sight or hearing—science would go forward to new conquests. Taking up the search where Galileo left it, Sir Isaac Newton of England was able to show mathematically that the same laws of motion observed on the earth were followed by the planets in the sky. He worked out the law of gravitation, which describes the way in which all bodies attract one another.

Newton, in terms of this law, could describe the orbits of all the known planets in exact figures and predict just where their regular movements would place them at any future time.

This made a great impression on learned men and they began to change their whole outlook on the universe. Instead of being mysterious, perhaps living beings, the planets were now viewed as great spheres moving majestically like a vast clock-work mechanism. They were so distant, vast, and mechanical that it seemed absurd to think that they had anything to do with little human lives below. Hence astronomers lost interest in astrology and its horoscopes, and gradually all educated men likewise abandoned it. After about 1700, doctors ceased consulting the stars in treating their patients.

This is not to say that there was no opposition to the new science. There was indeed something awesome, even disturbing, in the thought that man's earth was no longer the center of the universe. It seemed to make man less obviously the prime concern of his Creator. It is no wonder that some religious authorities thought it dangerous and heretical to teach that the earth, with all man's interests thereon, was but a speck in a cold, endless and indifferent space. Others were shocked at the repudiation of Aristotle's physics (which was not based on measurements), and claimed that the new discoveries were either false, or not really new, or at any rate useless.

Perhaps the whole matter would have stopped right there, with some arguing for the "experimental philosophy"—as the new science was called—and some against it, had it not been for the practical results. Soon it appeared that some of the discoveries actually were useful; they *did* make a difference. Practical inventions followed fast in the wake of pure science; Galileo himself invented a pendulum clock, from studying the pendulum as a special kind of moving body. (The principle is still used in present "grandfather clocks.") And the findings of astronomers were quite helpful in improving the art of navigation. But most spectacular was the work of physicists who, moving on from dynamics to the study of forms of matter, learned how to make air pumps as well as water pumps and so discovered much about the behavior of both liquids and gases.

From this came inventions like the thermometer and the barometer, which obviously were of practical value. Finally, in experimenting with steam, physicists revived the ancient Greek notion of a steam engine. Alexandrian scientists had made such a device long before the time of Christ, but failed to experiment with it and used it only as a toy. Now it was worked on more carefully, and by 1650 an Englishman set up a steam engine in London that could pump water higher than a church spire. Before 1700 machines of this type were actually in use to pump water out of mines. Steam power was to prove of greater labor-saving value than either animal, or wind, or ordinary water power. What wonders did not science hold for the future? More than any other single factor in the Renaissance, it promised a new kind of civilization.

Practical men were attracted by this utilitarian aspect of science. The influential and wealthy began in a small way to give it their support. When the more conservative universities opposed the "experimental philosophy," special academies devoted to it were founded in Rome, Paris, London and other centers. One of these, the Royal Society founded in London about 1660, has had a longer, continuous existence than has any other scientific body in the world today.

The churches, one should add, were gradually reconciled to the new viewpoints and religious opposition declined. This reconciliation was facilitated by a clearer distinction between the spheres of science and of religion. Descartes, a French mathematician, encouraged the view that science should give up the philosophical search for final truth with which it had been combined in medieval days. There should be no attempt to say *why* things ultimately came to be, for this was the task of religion and of philosophy. Science should simply describe Nature as accurately as possible, in the hope of aiding man to adapt himself to it more effectively.

This was much the view which had developed long before in Greece; but now scientists were in a far better position to pursue this goal than the Hellenes had been in the days of Hippocrates. Descartes was particularly hopeful of what *medical* science could do for mankind. "If human beings are to be perfected," he wrote (meaning in *this* world), "it will be through medicine that this will be accomplished." What changes had meanwhile occurred in medicine, that led to so optimistic and daring a conclusion?

Chapter VII

Medicine in a Changing World:

1500 to 1700

The sixteenth-century Renaissance witnessed in medicine the same trends as were to be observed in other natural sciences. There was the same revival of classical writers and a similar independence of these very authorities. Like the physicists, medical men benefited by the development of experimentation and other procedures. The connection between medicine and other sciences was close. All studies of Nature were known as "natural philosophy," and no sharp distinctions were made between physics, biology, and medicine. Galileo turned from one field to another as a matter of course. And since medicine was the one field to which a large profession was devoted, and in which a man could therefore make a living, the majority of scientists were physicians. Hence both modern chemistry and biology had their beginnings largely among medical men. It may be added that the discovery of new lands in America and in the East stimulated biological interests, because so many new plants and animals were revealed. This led to the establishment of the first botanical and zoological gardens. The "zoo" has been a popular place with city folk ever since.

Medicine necessarily shared the handicaps as well as the advantages of the period. Scientists were opposed at times by ecclesiastical authorities, Catholic and Protestant, who feared new views would lead to heresy. Sometimes this was because inquiring minds advanced unorthodox opinions. At other times it was because they clashed with religious officials in the actual practice of their profession, as when doctors who viewed mental disease as a medical problem ran afoul of religious doctrines on witchcraft. The Church also objected to the increasingly secular control of medical schools. When, for example, it forbade giving the degree to non-Christian students in Italy, the civil authorities in Venice ignored this and took the degree-granting function entirely into their own hands. Thus, certain scientists became the champions of the modern principle of freedom of thought.

One must remember, however, that the Church in other ways encouraged scientific work, so long as it did not conflict with theology. Some of the most famous physicians, among them Vesalius and Fracastoro, were patronized by popes and by such Catholic monarchs as Philip II of Spain. Frequently the chief obstacle to medical research, as in other sciences, came from a conservative majority within the profession itself. Those advancing new views had first to overcome an awe for Arabic authorities. And when this was achieved by the revival of original Greek classics, the veneration of Galen had to be surmounted. How extreme such conservatism could be is suggested by the aphorisms of a contemporary surgeon, one Michael Blondus, who declared, "It is more honorable to err with Galen or Avicenna than to be right with others;" and again, "It is better to die at the hands of a regular physician than to be saved by a quack."[23]

The last sentiment can be understood if the commonness of quackery is recalled. The fact that science was revealing new wonders, but that much in Nature remained inexplicable, tended to make people peculiarly credulous. The line between science and magic remained blurred. Alchemical quacks appeared in public squares, selling materials supposed to turn all things to gold; and at the same time other charlatans harangued the crowd about their wondrous cures. They employed clowns or musicians to attract a crowd and so originated the "medicine show," which survives even now in small American towns. The poor and ignorant depended largely on such quacks and on self-medication, or resorted to barbers for blood-letting and other routine services. Civil laws which required university training for physicians had been passed in Italy as early as the thirteenth century, and such regulations were common by 1500. But physicians

[23] Quoted in Victor Robinson, *The Story of Medicine*, p. 245.

were the elite group among medical practitioners and took care of only the upper classes.

Yet there were signs of professional progress: the flourishing medical schools of Italy, and later of northern lands; the prestige of learned physicians; the improved position of pharmacists and surgeons. Pharmacists already made up a respected guild. Their shops, following Arabian models, had first been set up in monasteries or in wealthy homes; but public pharmacies had appeared in Italy by 1250. Here physicians often interviewed their patients; indeed, it was not until the Renaissance that doctors transferred their chief public activities from these shops to the hospitals. Perhaps it was because of this earlier association that apothecaries dabbled in medical practice themselves, and their guilds provided much of the medical practice among those who could pay only moderate fees.

Surgeons also organized separate guilds. (Medieval physicians abandoned surgery because it involved work with the hands.) At times the surgeons combined with the barbers, for the latter performed routine bleeding, took care of skin conditions, and so on. Though unlearned, these barber-surgeons were sometimes skilful men. During the Renaissance, the revival of anatomical studies improved surgery, and this led leaders like Vesalius to demand that medicine and surgery should be combined once more. The prestige of surgeons slowly improved but their status remained inferior to that of physicians for a long period. Some rivalry developed between doctors and surgeons, as well as between doctors and apothecaries; and this was a source of professional confusion until after 1800.

The ideal which the public expected physicians to approach was changing in this period. During the Middle Ages the practitioner was at first expected to be a priest; later he was to be primarily a good and pious layman. During the Renaissance, it was assumed that he would be a "humanist;" that is, he should be a learned and cultivated person —a gentleman and a scholar. This was sufficient at the time, since it meant that he should keep his eyes open to the new intellectual world around him. Later, however, as experimental science advanced, something more came to be expected of him. The prominent physician should try new things, should investigate for himself. Once this stage was reached, the learning inherited from the Renaissance began to seem stuffy and pretentious. Molière and other literary lights ridiculed the pomposity and disputes of doctors, and delighted particularly in their quarrels during consultations.

Just because their art was so difficult and at the same time so vital to everyone, physicians could never escape public criticism of this sort. Mathematicians and artists had an easier time of it because most people were indifferent to their activities. The following lines from Molière's play, *L'Amour Médecin*, illustrate the contemporary burlesque of medical practice. Two doctors have been called to consult in the case of a certain layman's daughter. Enter the physicians:[24]

> *M. Thamès:* Sir, we have reasoned upon your daughter's distemper; and my opinion . . . is that it proceeds from a great heat of blood: so I'd have you bleed her as soon as you can.

> *M. Fonandrès:* And I say that her distemper is a putrefaction of humours . . . therefore I'd have you give her an emetic.

> *M. Thamès:* If you don't bleed your daughter out of hand, she's a dead woman.

> *M. Fonandrès:* If you do bleed her, she'll not be alive in a quarter of an hour hence.

All this left the family in some confusion. Finally it appeared that daughter had not been ill at all, and that the doctors had quoted Latin lore only to hide their ignorance of her condition.

Physicians might have retorted to Molière that the public itself was to blame for holding back their science. As in earlier periods, social and moral difficulties peculiar to medicine inhibited research. There was the age-old objection to human dissection. And in actual practice, cures were demanded in a hurry; so a doctor was tempted to jump at conclusions and claim all things for them. Otherwise the public would reward only the charlatan and the quack. Last but not least, the only way that doctors had to make a living was by daily practice, and this left them little time for original investigations.

Yet even in these respects the Renaissance brought improvements. The Church had long permitted occasional dissections of executed criminals, which usually meant two or three public performances a year at a given university. This was still the condition of things in northern Europe in 1500; but in sophisticated Italy the demands of both artists and medical men were breaking down aversion to ana-

[24] Quoted in Clendening, *Source Book of Medical History*, pp. 225, 226.

tomical studies. Vesalius, for example, found "subjects" scarce in Paris but had no such difficulty in Padua. One Italian physician claimed that he had examined a thousand cadavers. The same municipal authorities who permitted these investigations also supported their medical faculties financially, and so relieved the professors of some of the burdens of private practice. Such professional opportunities made possible the basic anatomical studies of the sixteenth century.

The New Anatomy

Ever since the Hellenistic Age there had been a persistent feeling that the secrets of health and disease, life and death, were concealed in the human body. Even if nothing had been found therein that really helped in treating the sick, there was still a curiosity about the mysteries of the body. Then, when humanists focused their attention on the natural man, this curiosity increased. Scholars wanted to see for themselves and not to rely simply on old authorities. And there was always the hope that useful as well as interesting discoveries might be made.

Even before Columbus made his great voyage to America, Italian anatomists were making more frequent dissections and were doing this work with their own hands. (The medieval method had been to read some fragment of Galen to a class, while an ignorant assistant tried to find the parts mentioned in the text.) The brilliant Leonardo da Vinci anticipated the whole spirit of the later Renaissance by discarding classical authorities, and based his investigations on some thirty dissections made by himself during the 1400's. Since he was one of the great artists of all time, his notebook sketches still afford some of the finest examples of anatomical art. Unfortunately his work was not published, and it was not until the next century that the real revolution in anatomy occurred.

The great name in this story is undoubtedly that of the Flemish anatomist Vesalius, who first studied and then taught at Padua. In 1543 he published, when only twenty-nine years old, his great *Fabrica* (The Fabric of the Human Body). Illustrated with magnificent engravings by the artist Calcar, this work completely replaced crude medieval concepts and also corrected some two hundred mistakes in the works of Galen. He demonstrated, for example, that there was no bone in the heart and that there were not two bones in the adult lower jaw—as Galen had assumed. More than this, he made an interesting discovery as to why the old Greek authority was fundamentally unreliable. As Vesalius himself said:[25]

> It now becomes obvious to us from the reborn art of dissection, [and] from diligent reading of the books of Galen . . . that he himself never dissected the body of a man who had recently died. . . . Nay, you may even find a great many things in his writings which he has not followed correctly in the apes; not to mention the manifold and infinite difference between the organs of the human body and the body of apes. . . .

In other words, the anatomy which had been taught throughout the Middle Ages had really been that of pigs and apes. No wonder that studies of this sort proved unreliable when applied to the body of man.

The text of Vesalius took up each general part in turn: the skeleton, the muscles, the vascular system, the abdomen, and so on. Of course, he made some errors and many smaller parts escaped his attention. These deficiencies were overcome by a number of great anatomists who followed him in the Italian universities in the 1500's, and in the medical centers of Holland, England, and Germany during the following century. Their names are often preserved in those of the organs they discovered; for instance, Fallopius found the Fallopian tubes and Eustachius, the Eustachian tube. These findings were sometimes denied by conservatives who held that if Galen seemed mistaken, it must be because the human body had changed since Roman times. But the arts of printing and of engraved illustrations spread the new anatomy throughout Europe and opposition gradually crumbled. By 1700 the gross anatomy of large organs and parts was known much as it is at the present time.

It did not take long in medicine, as in physical science, before pure research led to practical applications. In this instance, an improved knowledge of anatomy was of immediate value to surgeons. Barber-surgeons had picked up some trial-and-error skill but they needed also a systematic knowledge of body parts, which Vesalius could now give them. The advantage of putting folk experience and science together is well illustrated in the career of the famous French surgeon Ambroise Paré (1510–1590).

[25] Quoted in Clendening, *op. cit.*, p. 136.

Without university training and knowing no Latin, Paré learned in any empirical way he could—by accident, by trying out anything that occurred to him, by listening to "old women," and so on. Whereas Galileo had been a scholar who was not above learning from practical people, Paré *was* one of these people. Experience came to him while working in Paris hospitals and also on the battlefield. He revived the forgotten Roman device of the ligature, which greatly improved operative procedures. Bleeding no longer had to be stopped with the hot iron. He also abolished the practice of pouring boiling oil in gun-shot wounds, which had originated in the mistaken belief that these were poisoned by gun-powder. Turning his attention to obstetrics, which was naturally closely connected with surgery, he introduced podalic version and this was of great aid in unusual presentations. In much of his work, Paré was aided by his study of Vesalius. Surgery remained, after his time, limited chiefly to superficial operations, and not even practical experience taught the need for strictly aseptic procedures. But at least certain basic techniques like the use of the ligature were now known, and the belief that surgical infection (laudable pus) was desirable gradually declined.

Paré's contact with folk ideas was paralleled by that of the brilliant but eccentric German physician known as Paracelsus. The latter received regular medical training in Italy, but revolted violently against the ancient authorities. While Vesalius questioned politely, Paracelsus denounced and thundered. When appointed professor in a Swiss university, he is said to have publicly burned the books of Galen and other Greek classics. Such a gesture then seemed about as bad to physicians, as burning the Bible today would seem to good Christians. This medical rebel is sometimes compared to another German, Martin Luther, who at about the same time denounced established religious traditions. In any case, it is no wonder that Paracelsus was dismissed. He wandered back to his Swiss homeland, where he had been brought up in a mining region, and began to study the chemical processes involved in work with metals and minerals. He scorned neither miners nor alchemists and learned from both. So, too, he was constantly trying out his ideas in actual practice—entirely independently of the books.

Paracelsus emerged from all this with a new therapeutic doctrine; namely, that alchemists should cease trying to make gold and begin making medicines. He was convinced that, while Galen advocated vegetable drugs, the most potent were really the metals. He advocated the use of mercury, arsenic, and antimony, and a long debate ensued as to the relative merits of the two types of remedies. In the chemistry of metals and other materials, he held, would be found not only the secrets of drugs but also of the operations of the human body. (Here alchemy was finally coming to the professional surface, in the form of a physiological doctrine.) Paracelsus viewed the body as a sort of glorified chemical retort, activated by some mystical principle. Few men could understand such views at the time, but the chemical approach to physiology would not be forgotten.

Meanwhile, in the Italy which Paracelsus had abandoned, quite a different approach was being employed; there the new anatomy led directly to advances in physiology. This was in no way a revival of classical lore, for it will be recalled that Greek physiology was fanciful and confusing. Anatomists, as they observed each organ, became curious as to its uses. Vesalius himself was interested in physiological research and discussed vivisection of animals as a means to this end. Probably they would have gone no further than had the Greeks at this point, had it not been for the use of new scientific methods which were then coming into vogue. For while gross anatomy could be studied by simple observation, research in physiology required experiments, measurements, and the use of instruments to aid vision. One could describe the form of the brain by merely observing it, but without experiment its functions could never be determined.

The transition from anatomy to physiology, and the value of the new methods, is clearly indicated in the discoveries concerning the heart and blood vessels which ensued. Galen had declared that the vascular system centered in the liver, and that blood ebbed and flowed through the body via a septum between one side of the heart and the other. But anatomists now found that no such septum existed and this cast doubt on the whole theory. At the same time, the interest of physicists in air and water pumps suggested that the heart's motions might serve a pumping function.

About 1625 the Englishman Harvey—trained at Padua—finally solved the problem by experimenting and by measuring. He demonstrated experimentally on animals just how the blood flowed into the right auricle from the veins, thence to the right ventricle and out to the lungs—the contractions of the heart chambers providing the motive force. Then he traced the blood back from the lungs into the left auricle, to the left ventricle, and out into the arteries through the aorta. (Arteries had heretofore been said to hold only air and "vital spirits.") The valves of the heart and veins, already discovered by anatomists, were shown to check any possible back flow along these channels.

So simple an experiment as pressing a vein in the arm showed how the blood flowed towards the heart at that point, but could not be pressed backward because the valves in the vessel blocked any return. All the evidence pointed towards a continuous flow in one direction. That this flow must complete a circle was proved finally by simple measurements. The average volume of the blood which the heart held, before it pumped this into the aorta, was found to be about 2 ounces. With seventy-two beats per minute, this gave 72 x 2 or 144 ounces as forced out in that time. This meant 540 pounds an hour and several tons per day! Where could all this blood come from? Obviously the heart must be pumping the same blood round and round in a circle.

There was one uncompleted link in Harvey's chain of evidence. He could not see how the blood, having reached the end of the arteries, then found its way into small veins to begin the return journey to the heart. He simply assumed that it percolated through the peripheral tissues. At this point the instruments of observation "came in." The lens-grinders who had made the first telescopes, also contrived the earliest microscopes. An Italian anatomist, Malpighi, used one of these to examine blood vessels in the lung and other organs of frogs. In 1661 he announced that he had actually seen small arteries end in tiny vessels, which in turn led into the smallest of terminal veins. More than this, he had seen the blood flowing from arteries to veins through this network of capillaries. The picture of the circulation was now complete.

This demonstration, though at first opposed in the name of Galen and of the Arabians, made a great impression on the medical world. The mechanics of a bodily system had at last been described, much as the mechanics of a solar system had been outlined by astronomers. Perhaps physiology could be stated in terms of mechanical rather than chemical processes. Digestion could be viewed as a grinding procedure; muscular movements as the action of cords and levers. The

French philosopher Descartes began to write about "the animal machine." While much of this proved premature, since bodily functions were more intricate than could then be realized, an impulse was given to physiological research which resulted in considerable progress.

Development of the Understanding of Pathology

The value of anatomical studies was demonstrated in still another way during the Renaissance. In addition to advancing surgery and physiology, these led logically to the development of the medical science *par excellence;* namely, pathology. Greek pathology, like physiology, had been speculative in nature. There was the humoral doctrine which had come down from Hippocrates via Galen; and the opposing "Methodist" theory about tension and laxity in solid parts. And all this had led to a therapeutics of bleeding, sweating, and purging; either to rid the body of impure fluids, or to relax its tensions—according to which theory one preferred. (It must be admitted that most practitioners followed such theory and practice well into the nineteenth century.) But Renaissance anatomists, as early as the 1500's, began to picture disease processes in a more realistic way. This came about in the following manner.

Vesalius and others, in the course of their dissections, sometimes observed what seemed abnormal appearances in organs. Such "morbid anatomy" or pathology aroused their curiosity but at first they noted it only incidentally in their writings. As these observations grew in number, they received more attention; and a French physician, Fernel, set aside an entire section for pathology in a general text. He even described a case of appendicitis in 1567, with a clear account of post mortem conditions in the organ. A later French authority, Bonetus, published in 1679 a collection of all the observations on morbid phenomena which he could find in the earlier literature—a series which involved some three thousand cases. As a result of such accumulating evidence, a few men began to suspect that disease processes were not to be found in vague humoral conditions. They should be sought rather in abnormal changes in the structure of particular organs. This conception of a localized pathology, although not generally adopted before 1800, was destined in time to be of the utmost usefulness.

Development of Interest in the Means of Disease Transmission

While it is easy now, looking backward, to see the value of early research in physiology and in pathology, there were able physicians in the seventeenth century who doubted its value. Of what use was it to know that the blood circulated? Or how did it aid a man, ill with "consumption," to know that this was connected with tubercles in his lungs—as long as there was nothing the doctors could do about it? Early attempts to discover some practical application of physiology were disappointing. Blood was transfused from the circulation of animals to that of men, for example, but some of the subjects died. Hence it did not seem as if laboratory research had much to offer medical practice. In fact, each of these aspects of medical science went its own way for nearly two centuries thereafter, before laboratory men and clinicians found that they could be of mutual service.

Meanwhile, practitioners prided themselves upon being the practical men. Paracelsus had something of this clinical pride, but he became involved in mysticism. Quite different was Fracastoro, a contemporary Italian physician, who also observed the sick with an open mind but whose interests took him in a very different direction. While Paracelsus speculated on chemical and philosophical mysteries, Fracastoro stuck to the bedside evidence. It was during his life (1478–1553), just when leprosy was declining, that a serious and apparently new disease became endemic in Europe. This infection produced large sores (which led to the name "great pox" in contrast to smallpox) and was otherwise so dangerous and disfiguring that the public became alarmed. Fracastoro wrote a book about this plague, to which he gave the name of a mythological character—Syphilis. Some thought it a visitation for their sins and prayed for cures. Others said it had come from the New World with Columbus and historians are still debating this question.

In any case, Fracastoro was fascinated by the way in which he saw the same symptoms appearing in one person after another. It was as if some secret influence or poison, independent of the patients, was moving from one person to the next. This encouraged a view which had already been held of smallpox and measles; namely, that this was a disease distinct from all other illnesses. After describing syphilis, Fracastoro tried to define other special disorders. Here was the approach which the Greeks had rarely employed, for most of them had thought only of the patient and of his general condition. It did not identify a disease to say that a man was "bilious," or that he "had a fever." Only when it could be stated that he had a particular disease would specific diagnoses be possible. This was not the common practice in Fracastoro's time but he moved in that direction.

What interested him most, meantime, was the transmission of such diseases as syphilis, smallpox, and the plague. What was the poison involved? Since it seemed to enter a man and then to spread through this system, it acted as if it were alive and multiplied in the body. Hence the Italian physician spoke of the "seeds" of infection. The microscope was not yet available, so he never actually observed "germs" as we now understand the term. But he came close, as early as 1546, to the modern idea of infection by living organisms.

Fracastoro owed his insight in part to cumulative folk experience with leprosy and plague. This experience had convinced people that infections were contagious, despite the indifference of learned (classical) medicine to this view. Here again, as with Paré and Paracelsus, folk experience was coming to the professional surface and proving a valuable corrective to academic tradition. From common experience, too, Fracastoro derived the idea that diseases could be transmitted not only by contact between persons but also by infected clothing and other goods. "I call fomites," he observed, "such things as clothes, linen, etc., which although not themselves corrupt, can nevertheless foster the *essential seeds* of the contagion and thus cause infection."[26] It is hard to believe that this statement was made nearly four hundred years ago!

Fracastoro's approach to a theory of living contagion (*contagium vivum*) was supplemented a century later by the actual discovery of micro-organisms. Notable was the work of one Dutch lens grinder, Antony van Leeuwenhoek, who made his own microscopes and with the aid of remarkable vision amazed the world with his discoveries. Placing tartar from his teeth under the lens he saw, as had Galileo with his telescope, what human eyes had never seen before. Apparently clear water came alive with wriggling organisms. He even described bacteria in the 1660's! True, he did not formulate a real "germ theory" of disease. But this was done at about the same time by a German

[26] Quoted in Clendening, *op. cit.*, 107.

Jesuit Athanasius Kircher, who saw that these "little animals" might be Fracastoro's "seeds of contagion." Kircher searched for pathogenic germs in the bodies of plague victims and thought he found them; though in reality he probably saw nothing more than blood corpuscles.

The fear of syphilis and of bubonic plague led to increasing precautions against contagion. Old public baths were gradually closed, not to be reopened again until the nineteenth century. Bathing became a lost art. Measures once taken against leprosy, which had meantime retreated to Scandinavia, were applied to various epidemic diseases. There was no permanent isolation; but if a case of plague occurred in a house, the fear of "fomites" might lead to the burning of the whole building. Italian cities forced ships to ride in their harbors for forty days before landing goods, in order to insure that disease was not aboard. The Italian word for forty is *quaranto;* hence the word *quarantine* was applied to this practice when it was later adopted in England and other northern countries.

Fear of contagion was often carried to extremes between 1600 and 1800, while the preventive value of a cleanly environment was largely lost to sight. Later, after plagues declined, the sanitary ideal would be revived; and public hygiene would once more be torn between the relative merits of quarantine (against contagion) and of sanitary measures (against bad airs and waters).

Identification of Individual Diseases

The early interest in identifying diseases by their symptoms did not lead to any rapid progress in this direction. For one thing, the old humoral pathology continued to dominate medical minds; and if all illnesses were due to bad humors, it was only necessary to rid the body of these by bleeding and the like. Why bother trying to distinguish specific diseases if the treatment was always the same in any case? Here again, this speculative, humoral theory continued to retard clinical studies for centuries. The new pathology of local parts, already advanced by Fernel and Bonetus, might also have suggested specific diseases, but it was as yet only a minor note in medical thought.

Nevertheless, an interest in the clinical identification of distinct diseases never entirely disappeared. It was taken up again, for example, by the great English physician Sydenham in the seventeenth century. He became convinced that diseases were entities in themselves, apart from the patients who suffered from them, and that each disease had its own history. Thus an epidemic disease varied in virulence from one period to another. He carefully described a number of different diseases; for example, gout, dysentery, measles, and so on. Doctors, he held, should not simply observe patients in a general way but should study these diseases as such. If one could diagnose each case, that is, tell just what form of illness was present, then perhaps he could look for the special cause or treatment needed for that particular complaint. In other words, specific diagnosis might lead to specific therapy.

Here was a thought largely foreign to Greek or medieval medicine but one which was big with possibilities for the future. Its significance was already apparent, indeed, in the case of syphilis. The specific identification of this disease had made possible specific treatment with mercury—one of Paracelsus' metals—and this had proved of some value.

Unfortunately, Sydenham could see no way of identifying diseases except by symptoms. Except in certain striking infections like smallpox, symptom combinations were endless and were apt to be confusing. Later doctors found this out to their cost. It never occurred to Sydenham that the new localized pathology might aid him here. Why not check up on a disease by seeing what happened inside the body as well as outside? But this thought escaped him; perhaps because he was a bedside observer and gave little heed to the anatomists. So clinical and pathological research—bedside and death-house observations—each continued to go its own way for another century, before they were finally brought together to make possible modern diagnoses.

Therapeutic Concepts

Meanwhile, Sydenham's efforts to observe cases and to experiment with treatments led him to advocate new ways of handling the sick. After all, therapeutics needed to be rescued from ancient errors just as much as did anatomy. Tradition said that those suffering from fevers (having bad humors) should have these sweated out of them under heavy coverings in closed rooms. But Sydenham found that patients fared better with light clothing and with fresh air. The English philosopher Locke was so impressed with these independent, practical procedures that he wrote, "I wonder that, after the pattern

Dr. Sydenham has set them of a better way, men should return to the romance way of physic."[27]

But once again the views of a superior man were ignored by the rank and file of practitioners. There were as yet few medical societies and no medical journals, and even with printed books it was hard to overcome the professional traditions of centuries. Most physicians continued to accept the humoral pathology and to follow such traditional treatments as bleeding, purging, and the use of all sorts of bizarre, complicated and repulsive drugs. The first pharmacopoeias, published in Italy in the 1500's and in England about 1650, eliminated some of the more complicated Arabian compounds. But these manuals still contained such remedies as crab's eyes, animal dung, human sweat, oil of puppies boiled with earth worms, and so on *ad nauseam*.

In Sydenham's own time, King Charles II of England became mortally ill, and the account of the treatments to which he was subjected is still preserved. Among other things, his majesty was bled from the right arm and the left shoulder; was given emetics, purgatives, and an enema made of thirteen mineral and vegetable substances; a blister was raised on his scalp, and a sneezing powder given to purge the brain of phlegm—the old humoral notion. A plaster of pitch and pigeon dung was placed on his feet. Then he drank a concoction of melon seeds, slippery elm, cherry water, extract of lily of the valley, peony, lavender, pearls dissolved in vinegar, nutmeg, and cloves. In this was included as a last resort some extract of human skull. Finally the King died, actually apologizing to his doctors for being so long in the process!

The strange and complicated drugs prescribed for Charles II were largely inherited from medieval and even more ancient traditions. Old concoctions recalled from Roman times were supplemented by weird doses whose appeal was to superstition and to credulity. The "extract of human skull," secured from crossroad gibbets, is a case in point. But the seventeenth century also witnessed in pharmacy some advances of both a professional and scientific nature. The Apothecaries Guild had been united with the Grocers Guild in London during the 1500's, apparently because they sold some things in common. In other parts of Europe, as in Italy, the pharmacists had long sold various goods

[27] Quoted in Knud Faber, *Nosography*, 2 ed., Paul B. Hoeber, Inc., (N.Y., 1930), 16, 17.

besides drugs in their shops. (This anticipated the tendency of the present American drugstore to function as a small department store.) But such an arrangement had its disadvantages, so that the English Apothecaries Guild appealed to James I about 1620 for separation from the Grocers. The King granted this on the ground that the latter were merchants but the former a "mystery"—that is, a profession.

So encouraged, the Apothecaries built their own hall and set up their own laboratory, botanic garden, and dispensary. Gradually they gave their apprentices certain elements of medical training; and eventually they came to compete with physicians in general practice. Meantime the Guild issued the *London Pharmacopoeia,* which King James ordered every apothecary in England to follow. This was not only the first one issued in English, but the first to be officially adopted by a national government—an interesting example of "state medicine." Many other municipal pharmacopoeias were issued during the 1600's. While these contained all the nonsense noted above, a few really valuable drugs came into use during this century. Some were discovered by alchemists, such as Glauber's salts (sodium sulphate). Others had been long known in a vague way but were first clearly defined and defended by physicians in this era. Sydenham's use of a tincture of laudanum is a good illustration of this. The most useful remedies were those recently discovered in America. Such Latin American plant-products as cascara, jalap (a powerful purgative), and cinchona bark, all came into more or less permanent use.

The latter was at first known as "Jesuit's Bark" in England, since Jesuits had been active in introducing it via Spain from Peru. It had long been known to Indian folk medicine, and proved to be a specific against malaria—one of the first truly specific drugs ever discovered. As such, it was a real boon to millions in both Europe and America who suffered from various forms of "chills and fevers." About two hundred years later, in 1825, the active principle of "quinine" was isolated from the bark by French chemists.

Other American vegetable products, such as tobacco, were thought to be medically useful in the 1600's but have long since been restricted to less serious uses. It is interesting, incidentally, to learn that lemonade was prized as a medicine because of its anti-scorbutic properties, and that it was sometimes used in frozen form. In other words, lemon sherbet was taken seriously as a medicine. So, too, was maple sugar.

The taking of such pleasant materials as tobacco, lemonade, and maple sugar may have compensated somewhat for the more revolting doses which were common at the time. Tobacco, however, was not introduced without a valiant struggle against the "vile weed." King James I himself wrote a book against it, and medical as well as moral opposition to its use continues at the present time.

Treatment of the Insane

Still more depressing than the story of general practice, is the account of the treatment of the insane. In no period were the mentally ill dealt with so cruelly as in the sixteenth and seventeenth centuries. Classical physicians, as noted before, had viewed mental disturbances as one type of disease and treated them accordingly. A similar view persisted with some medieval physicians and the insane had been cared for in the early hospitals. But the tendency in the later Middle Ages was to view such people as "possessed" of a demon or even by the Devil himself. For centuries the clergy tried to exorcise such spirits out of the afflicted.

By 1500 a more severe attitude became apparent. It was asserted that "possessed" individuals were witches who had voluntarily submitted to the Devil, receiving in return malevolent powers to injure their neighbors. It was therefore necessary to destroy witches in order to protect the community. Two German friars, Sprenger and Kraemer, preached this doctrine with savage effectiveness in the late 1400's, and finally persuaded Church authorities to give it their sanction. In this way the treatment of mental illness was taken out of the hands of physicians and turned over to ecclesiastic and civil officials. Some physicians, it must be admitted, concurred, and reconciled old humoral interpretations with the theological view. There ensued veritable epidemics of witch hunting, in which hundreds of thousands of persons— many of them demented—were tortured and burned. Not all of those executed were insane. But nearly all the insane, because of their strange behavior, were suspected of witchcraft. There is no more tragic chapter in the history of Christianity.

No simple explanation can be given for this vast delusion. Centuries of preoccupation with the relation of the soul to the forces of evil, and especially with the dangers of sex, had much to do with it. Women were viewed by ascetic theologians as a constant temptation;

and it cannot be overlooked that the witchcraft literature was saturated with sex and that women were the chief victims. It is also true that certain popular manias were widespread during the 1400's, and leaders honestly feared that the Devil was abroad. From this angle, the witchcraft persecutions were a sort of deluded public health movement. Then the Reformation struggles, which promoted bigotry in both religious camps, aroused a desire to stamp out witchcraft as a form of heresy. Protestants vied with Catholics in a crusade of extermination.

There was, finally, a certain amount of malice and hypocrisy involved. There always is in such widespread upheavals. Men found it convenient to accuse their enemies. Certain clergymen and judges apparently took sadistic pleasure in the examinations and tortures. Public leaders found in the hysteria a useful rationalization of their own conduct. When Henry VIII of England wearied of Queen Anne Boleyn, he claimed that he had been seduced by witchcraft into the marriage, and "cited as proof that the Lord had not allowed them to have any male issue."[28]

It is only fair to add that some church authorities were reluctant to accept the extreme doctrines of Sprenger and Kraemer. Other leaders expressed cautious doubts even at the height of the hysteria. While such medical men as Paré and Fernel believed firmly in witches, the French essayist Montaigne ridiculed the whole idea. Inspired by the critical outlook of Renaissance science, moreover, certain physicians protested that mental disease *was* a medical problem and that theological interference therein was uncalled for and dangerous. A German doctor, Johann Weyer, investigated cases and showed how they were susceptible to purely natural interpretations. (His statements remind one of the Hippocratic writing "On the Sacred Disease," in which a Greek physician had rejected theological explanations of epilepsy nearly two thousand years before.) To express such views required courage in the 1500's, and they did not check the madness at the time. The mentally ill continued for two centuries to be in some danger and were denied even attempts at medical treatment. But Weyer's work foreshadowed an outlook which later would be widely adopted, as science advanced and theological zeal declined.

[28] Quoted in Gregory Zilboorg and George W. Henry, *A History of Medical Psychology*, New York, W. W. Norton and Co., Inc., 1941, p. 153.

In summing up the early modern period, 1500–1700, one has to balance much that was backward against certain advances of a most basic nature. The ordinary practice of the times was conservative and even reactionary. Most physicians did not depart from what Locke called "the romance way of physic" nor would they for a century to come. The neglect of the insane was particularly depressing. Yet medical science had finally awakened after a millennium of medieval slumber. New outlooks and new methods led to discoveries which would one day benefit practice as well as theory. Medicine, for all its shortcomings, was pointed in promising directions as it entered the eighteenth century.

Chapter VIII

Impact of Secular Trends on
Hospitals and Nursing:
1500 to 1700

The sad state of routine medical practice during the early modern era was paralleled at times by deplorable conditions in hospitals and in nursing. Indeed, the phrase "Dark Age of Nursing" has been applied to the period from 1600 to as late as 1850. The economic and cultural advances of the Renaissance brought little improvement in hospital services, and in some respects these services deteriorated during the transition to a new age.

In the first place, the failure of medical research to improve ordinary practice was—in a negative sense—a factor in holding back hospital progress. Had science provided any improved treatments, this might have aroused interest in nursing and bettered its status. As it was, physicians only continued their dosings and bleedings, and expected of nurses simply the custodial care which they had always given their charges. Hence the relation of medical science to nursing remained unchanged.

Moreover, while science neither advanced nor retarded nursing, other factors exerted a definitely adverse influence. When the whole tone of European life became increasingly secular, such religious institutions as hospitals had difficulty in adjusting themselves to the change. Evidences of the new outlook, such as the growing power of the State and the increasing cultivation of worldly business and amusements, were apparent in Catholic as well as in Protestant lands. Although the Reformation struggle revived religious zeal, it did not halt the secular trend in the long run.

Under these circumstances, great folk were less inclined to found hospitals or to serve in them than had been the case in earlier days. They were too busy with other matters; and, besides, the civil government could take care of these things. The middle classes now had more money; let them support charities by contributions or taxes. Such views developed slowly, but that was the tendency over a long period. At the same time, some of those in charge of hospitals were affected by the same worldliness and neglected their charges while tending to their own comfort. Signs of trouble had been obvious even before the Reformation.

In some small English institutions, for instance, patrons, wardens, and attendants exploited their trust for selfish advantage. Patrons poached on hospital funds, kings made grants (corodies) which permitted their friends to do the same, and wardens neglected the sick while they and the brethren lived on the endowments. To make matters worse, beggars and malingerers imposed on such places as were trying to do their duty well.

Meanwhile, the income of institutions declined over the years and this made for internal decay. St. Leonard's of York, for example, received in 1370 an income of about £1,300 and cared for 224 patients. By 1409 the funds had fallen to £546, and within another half century it was providing for only about 125 inmates. In extreme cases buildings deteriorated, equipment was sold, and depravity reigned in the households. Robert Copland, in a fifteenth-century poem written when the English language was beginning to take modern form, protested that:

> I have sene at sondry hospytalles
> That many have lyen dead without the walles
> And for lacke of socour have dyed wretchedly
> Unto your foundacyon I thynke contrary

That bad conditions were widespread is indicated in a statute of 1414 for the reform of English hospitals. This declared, "Many hospitals . . . be now for the most part decayed, and the goods and profits of the same . . . spent to the use of others, whereby many men and women have died in great misery for default of aid."[29]

No doubt some of this deterioration was due to factors which affect old establishments in general. The zeal of the founders was long since past. What pioneers had struggled for, later generations took for granted. The certainty of endowment income attracted those who wanted an easy life and this lowered the quality of staff and personnel. The temptation to live on the income remained a demoralizing factor in some places well into the eighteenth century. When the Pennsylvania Hospital was founded in Philadelphia about 1750, for example, the first gift of real estate was made to it by a local German who warned against the misuse of such endowments. He declared that in Germany he had frequently seen hospital officials living on the funds they were supposed to devote to the poor.

In the normal course of events, when old institutions decay, new movements replace them with young and virile organizations. But during the Renaissance, reviving secular activities diverted interest away from hospital endowments. Then came the Reformation and this produced further difficulties. The Reformation, it is true, had no direct effect on hospitals in Catholic countries, and some hospitals survived in Protestant lands. Most of the larger ones in England, Germany, and Scandinavia continued to operate, or resumed operations after a short interval. But many small institutions were closed in Protestant countries when the nursing orders were suppressed, and this action also led to certain modifications in the large city establishments.

The most serious consequences occurred in England. Here Henry VIII, after his break with Rome, suppressed all the orders and confiscated the property of some six hundred charitable endowments. Many of these were still devoted to one form or another of "poor relief"; and beggars, orphans, and old people suffered as much as did those who were acutely sick. Eventually, the civil government had to take over general public relief, and during Elizabeth's reign a regular "Poor Law" system was worked out for this purpose. Thereafter, the sick poor in small towns gravitated into the "almshouses" which were set up by Poor Law Boards and were supported by local taxation.

[29] Quotations from R. M. Clay, *English Medieval Hospitals*, London, 1909, pp. 212, 226.

This arrangement was more systematic than that of the old Church establishments and may at first have been more efficient than outworn medieval provisions. But state charity, lacking the idealism of the better church organizations, acquired a stigma that offended the very classes who needed it. And in due time public charity became not only cold and indifferent but scandalously inefficient. The phrase "over the hill to the poorhouse" still conveys unhappy implications.

As far as the history of nursing is concerned, the fate of the large English hospitals was more important than was that of the small ones. The former were the ones which limited their work to the care of the sick and in them lay the future of both medicine and nursing. Speaking generally, those maintained by monasteries or private patrons were permanently closed; while those supported by towns or by cathedrals survived. Developments can be best observed in the case of the London establishments. The three general hospitals, St. Mary's, St. Thomas', and "St. Bartylmew's" were closed about 1538, and the first was never reopened. What subsequently happened is well illustrated in the case of the last-named institution.

When St. Bartholomew's was ordered closed, its services to the city were so well known that citizens soon petitioned to have it continue. The authors of this petition declared that there were now "miserable people lying in the streets offending every clean person passing by the way with filthy and nasty savours." Within a few years (1544) the King was practically forced to reopen "Bart's" and to return to it some endowment.

In rededicating the hospital, Henry posed as a founder and his portrait still ornaments a window in the Great Hall. His proclamation on this occasion was piously worded and again revealed the necessity for his action. First he observed that "The poor, aged, sick, low, and impotent people . . . being infected with divers great and horrible sicknesses and diseases" were lying about or begging in the streets of London. Then he added magnanimously:[30]

> His Highness of his bountiful goodness and charitable mind
> moved with great pity for . . . the said poor . . . , and for the
> avoiding of the great danger and infection which daily doth
> and may ensue to his loving subjects by reason of the . . .

[30] Quoted in Sir D'Arcy Power, *A Short History of St. Bartholomew's Hospital, 1123–1923*, London, 1923, p. 31.

> horrible diseases of the same sick and low people . . . is pleased
> to grant to the Mayor and Citizens of London and their
> successors forever the late hospital of St. Bartholomew.

Several points in this statement are worth noting, in addition to the apparent hypocrisy of the noble Henry. First, observe the mixture of motives, part pity, part fear. The citizens were offended by horrible sights and were fearful of contagion. This last was an expression of folk beliefs about contagion—beliefs then being raised to a science by Fracastoro in Italy. Such fear not only led to the support of hospitals but later would be a potent factor in promoting all public health procedures. Second, it will be observed that the King did not turn the hospital over to the Church of England but rather confirmed its civil (secular) character.

In the reorganization which followed, "Bart's" did not become a strictly municipal establishment. It was governed rather by the Mayor and by a self-perpetuating board of its own. In this way it was closely associated with public service but was not under the direct control of the city government. In this respect, it later served as a model for the first hospitals in the American Colonies.

Curiously enough, all through the period when St. Bartholomew's was officially closed, patients stayed in the buildings. Some attendants must have remained to look after them. After the reorganization, five "sisters" were appointed to tend the sick and one of these was to serve as supervisor or "matron." Obviously, much of the nursing tradition carried on. Not only were the attendants called "sisters," though they were lay people, but it was provided that they should continue to wear a special habit. To this day most English nurses use the same title. The matron was supposed to take the place of a prioress or superior, the other "sisters" that of the nuns. The latter were even ordered to "avoid and shun the conversation and company of all men." Clearly, they were expected to live and labor somewhat as had a medieval, secular order.

It is difficult to determine just how far the sisters, either before or after the Reformation, carried on the nursing routine. On the one hand, we are told that they not only did actual nursing but also all menial tasks as a matter of devotion. The directions given the sisters of St. Bartholomew's in 1544 declared that they should "do their duty unto the poor in making of the beds and keeping their wards as also in washing and purging their unclean clothes and other things." Elsewhere they were directed to keep the poor patients "sweet and clean"—which must have been quite an achievement in some cases— and to give them "their meats[31] and drinks after the most honest and comfortable manner." If all this was not enough to keep them busy, the matron should set them "to spinning or doing of some other manner of work that may avoid idleness and be profitable to the poor of this House."[32]

On the other hand, there were never enough sisters in "Bart's" to take care of all the patients and servant-attendants must have been present. Little was said of them, perhaps because they were just taken for granted. By the 1600's a class of "women helpers" was clearly defined, some of whom eventually became "sisters." They were half nurses, half servants—in terms of modern distinctions—and the relation of the sister to them suggests the office of a floor or ward supervisor. Eventually the "helpers" became known as nurses. Other types of workers in the English hospital of 1600, such as the "night watchers" who came in when needed, have no present counterparts except that night duty occupies the same hours.

Sisters, and to a lesser degree the helpers or nurses, were expected to observe a rather rigid discipline. This may be traced in part to the vows taken by nursing groups before the Reformation and was considered necessary for the sake of morale. It has also been suggested that the discipline followed in military nursing orders had influenced general hospital procedures. Perhaps this example encouraged distinctions in rank among hospital personnel which have survived in a lessened degree to our own time. The sisters at St. Bartholomew's were directed to be obedient to the matron who was their "chief governess and ruler." They could not go out of the woman's ward (the old dormitory of the nuns, opening off the patients' hall) after seven in winter or nine in summer. Should they witness anything questionable in others they must report it to the matron or governors (Board), "and to no other person neither shall you talk or meddle therein any further."[33]

[31] The old English "meats" referred to various foods, and is preserved in such a modern term as "sweet meats."
[32] *Ibid*, 39.
[33] *Ibid*., 40, 41.

Various steps were taken to improve St. Bartholomew's in the course of the reorganization. Three surgeons were appointed in 1549, with salaries, to attend regularly upon the patients; and by 1568 a physician was also in attendance. The greater need for surgeons may be ascribed to the prevalence of skin conditions and injuries among the poor who sought shelter in this period. New officials were added to the staff in the person of "beadles" whose duty is was to police the buildings and the surrounding neighborhood. Vagrants and malingerers were to be kept out, and at the same time those in real need were to be brought in from the streets. These officials were partly attached to the hospital, partly to the police authority of the local government.

In all these matters, this London hospital was expected to carry on much as it had always done. There was even provision, through the vicar of the local Anglican parish, for the spiritual welfare of patients and personnel. Yet the reorganization led in time, perhaps unintentionally, to certain important changes in St. Bartholomew's and other city hospitals in England. First, the institutions gradually became more secular in atmosphere. While some had been owned by towns before the Reformation, their operation had been in the hands of religious communities. Now the latter had ceased to exist. Hence actual management came into the hands of the lay governors or trustees. The vicar might hold services but could not take the place of a former prior or superior. Neither could the steward, who continued to handle business affairs and who was analogous to the superintendent of a modern hospital.

To put it in another way, the Church of England did not retain the influence over hospital services that had long been exerted by the Catholic authorities. The Anglican Church did not lose all interest in hospitals or other welfare organizations. Parishes continued to support local charities. The Bishop of London urged Henry's successor, Edward VI, to increase the support of hospitals in the diocese. In consequence, Christ's Hospital for children was founded in 1553 and St. Thomas' was revived a few years later. But lacking monastic orders at this time, the Anglicans necessarily left management and nursing to lay personnel.

Such management raised serious questions. In a time when medical science required no training for nurses beyond what could be picked up through experience, nursing was bound to be a matter of difficult and often unpleasant routine. If this were true of the sisters in charge of a hall, it was even more true of "helpers" who did the work both of nurses and servants. Under the old régime, religious devotion had ennobled this toil and had made it seem worthwhile. But could such idealism be maintained with a lay personnel? If not, would the one-time service of devotion descend into mere drudgery?

This danger had always existed but it became greater when nursing shifted to sisters and helpers who took no vows. Good women, some of whom were inspired by idealism, doubtless served after the reorganization. But superior persons were less likely to enter the service when it no longer had a religious character. Membership in a nursing order brought with it dignity and a possibility of recognition. And in recent times, in contrast, nursing has been so advanced by medical progress that it has become professional in nature. But for more than three centuries after the Reformation, secular nursing involved no career whatever. No wonder that the better types of women tended to abandon it.

Meantime, women of some sort had to be found for service in hospital wards. And what women would want such a job, with its poor pay, confining discipline, and unpleasant routine? Obviously, chiefly those who because of age, poverty, or ignorance could get nothing better. Here was a situation which slowly and insidiously undermined the nursing services of the ensuing centuries. The situation was not peculiar to England or even to Protestant countries, as will be noted later, but it became most evident in English institutions.

Certain of the changes, made during the reorganization of "Bart's" and of other English hositals, reflected the economic trends of the time. Since a capitalistic or business economy was then emerging, more and more people were being compensated for services in money, rather than being "paid in kind" or just given "a living" on lands as in feudal days. This meant that sisters and nurses in English hospitals had to be paid wages as employees. And in order to raise funds for this purpose, the governors (boards of trustees) began raising a little money from the patients. These people were required, for example, to deposit burial fees before being admitted. Even though these were returned in cases of recovery, some hardship was involved for the very poor. The matrons, beadles, and porters also expected tips or small fees for their services. Hospital care thus ceased to be entirely benevolent in nature.

As already suggested, the reorganization of city hospitals throughout England followed trends similar to those in London. Much the same thing can be said of large hospitals in other Protestant countries. City establishments were necessarily retained but taken out of the hands of the suppressed orders. Smaller hospitals on the Continent, however, were not so suddenly or systematically closed as in England. In Denmark and Sweden the leper hospitals, perhaps because of surviving need there, were retained and in time became general isolation or pest-houses. In the former country Franciscan friaries, which had usually ministered to some sick persons, were frequently turned into small hospitals. In some of the German cities an effort was made to compensate for the loss of religious houses by setting up municipal infirmaries in each part of town. These were plainly marked so that the poor could locate them, and the civil authorities appointed nursing attendants—both men and women—to serve in them. During the transitional period, women who had served as Beguines were encouraged to take over this function.

In Scandinavia and in some German principalities, moreover, the Lutheran State Church continued to support hospitals. Orders of Lutheran sisters served in these institutions, which thus retained more of the pre-Reformation atmosphere than did the English hospitals. There were also other indications that nursing was taken more seriously in Germany. One of these may be mentioned at this point; namely, the appearance of the first nursing manuals. As early as 1574, for example, one Jacob Oetheus published in Germany a general work on the care of the sick. He stressed in this the virtues usually expected of attendants, the importance of following the doctor's orders, and the need for taking the doctor's place if emergencies demanded this. Expressing a Protestant viewpoint, Oetheus recommended the employment of married men and of older widows as nurses. He expected that married men would observe the proprieties, and that widows would not be diverted by obligations to husbands or children.

Control of Hospitals

Even before the Reformation, there had been signs of trouble in hospitals on the Continent as well as in England. Difficulties arose in large city institutions where increasing numbers of poor overburdened the nursing facilities. Sisters and Brothers often depended upon convalescents for help, and this and other factors led to some demoralization. Municipal authorities, hearing complaints, investigated and began to exert some control. As early as the fourteenth century, the larger hospitals in Italy and Germany were thus taken into municipal hands, and during the sixteenth century the same process ensued in France. This secular trend was a gradual one in Catholic cities, as compared to the sudden and extreme secularization which occurred in Protestant countries, but it moved in the same direction.

The conflict involved between religious and civil authorities was especially protracted in France. It always centered on the nursing factor, so that the Brothers and Sisters were in a sense caught between the contending powers. An illustration of the extremes to which the struggle was sometimes carried is afforded by the Hôtel-Dieu in Paris, which was under the control of the Cathedral of Notre Dame.

Conditions at the Hôtel-Dieu became bad in the 1400's and remained so for several centuries. The Augustinian Sisters, because of overwork, kept convalescents around to assist in their labors. This weakened discipline and nursing; and civil officials objected both for this reason and on grounds of economy. The latter also held that Sisters were encouraged to give so much time to religious matters that they neglected the patients. The Parliament of Paris passed edicts to regulate routine and limited the number of Sisters who could serve. These rules met with resistance by Brothers and Sisters, who were sometimes supported by local priests. When new masters or supervisors were appointed by the government, actual riots broke out within the hospital in which the convalescents joined. Even the canons of Notre Dame, hurrying to quell the disturbance, were refused admittance.

Repeated difficulties finally led King Louis XII, in 1505, to take control of the hospital from the canons of the Cathedral and to invest it in civil appointees. There ensued nearly three more centuries of friction between the civil directors on the one hand, and the Sisters and clergy on the other. The former accused the Sisters of hiring old women to do the night watching, of still spending too much time on religious matters, and of general insubordination. The latter answered that most of the difficulties were due to excessive economy and to a lack of adequate staff. A new note was introduced in the 1600's, when

162

physicians began to complain that their orders were not carried out in the wards. Eventually, in 1692, the directors introduced paid servants to take the place of the convalescents, and extended this service to housekeeping as well as to the wards. In this way hired help came in which later proved of an inferior sort, but meanwhile these persons were independent of the Sisters and their presence contributed to secular control.

It is difficult to weigh the pros and cons of this long controversy. Much of the trouble undoubtedly resulted from the parsimony of civil directors. On the other hand, conditions had become bad under the old order; and when Sisters resisted the influence of physicians they were opposing a demand for truly medical care. Eventually, in the late 1700's, they were ordered to turn over the acceptance and discharge of patients to the doctors. Taking a final stand on the ground that they were responsible only to Church authorities in such matters, they were overruled by the civil directors. What was really going on here was a long struggle between the medieval religious tradition and the modern trend toward secular administration. The three main stages of the process were the appointment of civil directors, the employment of paid servants, and finally the establishment of professional medical control.

Meantime, the problem presented by village institutions in Catholic countries was of a somewhat different nature. Shifts in population, the decline of leprosy, falling income and other factors left many small places useless or without funds. Certain groups administering them became careless or exploited the endowments for their own purposes. In France, where the royal power was developing rapidly, monarchs became convinced that these institutions would be better managed if taken out of the hands of local lords (patrons) or clergy and placed under civil control. Thus Charles IX, in 1561, ordered that village hospitals should be placed under the administration of substantial citizens in each community. He also followed the suggestions of humanist scholars in ordering better medical attendance and more equitable distribution of funds.

By the end of the Reformation era, then, the administration of many French hositals had come under the same middle-class, lay control as developed in Protestant countries. Other parallels between Catholic France and Protestant England will be noted shortly, in order to point out that some of the changes here were common to all commercial countries and not primarily due to religious differences. The latter factor does appear, however, in the continuation of religious nursing in the French as well as in other Catholic institutions. Where hospitals came under lay direction on the Continent, moreover, they were usually under government control rather than the private administration common in England.

Development of Religious Nursing Orders

The religious struggles of the Reformation had no direct effect upon hospitals in such Catholic lands as Spain and Italy. When the Council of Trent met from 1545 to 1564, however, it undertook the reform of various practices in the Catholic Church as a whole. The challenge of Protestantism—or of secularism—was to be met.

One problem which received attention was laxity or inefficiency in the complicated system of religious orders. Some of these bodies were regular and some secular in character. Some were large organizations reaching all over Western Europe, others small and local in nature. One group might be devoted to a contemplative life, another primarily to social service. In the latter category lay such diverse functions as the support of education, special homes or refuges, and the care of the sick poor.

The general result of the Council's deliberations on the orders was a series of regulations intended to "tighten up" morale and discipline. Stricter vows were required of old orders, and new ones were not accepted unless these standards were met. For nearly three hundred years after 1550, papal approbation was refused for any monastic groups save those willing to undertake permanent vows of celibacy and of obedience. As these vows required an enclosed life, freedom to engage in nursing became very restricted. Emphasis necessarily shifted, within the regular orders, towards the contemplative ideal. As had sometimes occurred before the Reformation, however, this led to the founding of pious associations taking no perpetual vows and therefore not restricted to an enclosed life. The need for nursing continued, and if old orders like the Poor Clares could no longer supply it, others must take their place.

One of the more important of such new orders was that founded by a Portuguese soldier, Juan Ciudad, about the time of the Reformation. This was originally a group of laymen organized to nurse men in the hospitals. Somewhat later they took a rule which did not prevent such activities and extended their work throughout the Continent as the Brothers of Charity. Usually they established their own house adjacent to a hospital, and went back and forth in the course of their duties. By the eighteenth century, they were probably the best known nursing Brothers (*baumherzigen Brüder*) in Catholic Germany.

The organization of new men's orders, with the zeal usually characteristic of youthful societies, was a desirable development. For it must be remembered that, with certain exceptions to be noted later, women were usually not permitted to nurse in men's halls. The whole trend in the later medieval Church had been towards a strict separation of the sexes in all ecclesiastical institutions; and as late as 1800 it was usually considered bad taste, if not actually immoral, to place sisters in male wards.

In contrast to this, women began to nurse in men's halls in some of the Protestant countries soon after the Reformation. In England, for example, "women helpers" took over the care of both sexes. Just why such a new departure occurred there is not easy to explain. Perhaps the English helpers were considered a hardened lot who could "take it." A more complimentary interpretation would be to say that Protestantism became less ascetic in its ideals and therefore less insistent on sex segregation. In any case, hospital authorities in Catholic Europe long opposed the English procedure as inconsistent with their own standards. Male orders therefore continued to occupy an important place in the Catholic nursing picture.

Yet the activity of women in nursing became quite marked in Catholic lands after the Reformation. All told, more than one hundred female orders or congregations—many without rigid vows—have been founded since that era for this purpose. Some had so brief an existence that very little is known of them. But the cumulative figures are impressive, and certain of the new organizations proved of lasting importance. Notable was the organization of the Sisters of Charity by St. Vincent de Paul.

The latter was one of those rare spirits who, as did St. Francis before him and John Howard in a later day, combined sympathy for the poor with a genius for organized reform. After being trained as a Franciscan, St. Vincent de Paul was captured by Barbary pirates and was sold as a slave. He thereby became familiar with the sufferings of this class. Later he succeeded in returning to Paris, where he saw much of the privations of the poor in a large town. He was appalled, for example, by the number of infants left at church doors or otherwise abandoned, and succeeded in establishing two of the first foundling asylums for these unfortunates. His interest in the proper care of small children anticipated a widespread infant welfare movement which had important consequences in the next century.

St. Vincent also became familiar with the sufferings of the sick poor, while assisting the Brothers who served in the Charité Hospital in Paris. Upon removing to a country parish in 1617, he organized there a society of ladies who agreed to visit the sick in their own homes in order to provide both nursing and religious encouragement. As far as nursing was concerned, their activities were partly analogous to those of later visiting nurses; and this extension of services into homes is of interest in itself. One cannot say that this had never been done before, even in the medieval period; and it certainly was a feature of the work of the early Christian deaconesses. But it became, in the century which followed St. Vincent, a regular feature of the work of certain communities.

The services of this early group of charitable women were so well received that similar societies were established in other towns. In 1629 one was organized in Paris under the leadership of the remarkable Mlle. Le Gras. Here it was found that the ladies were inclined to send their servants to do the actual nursing; and in consequence numbers of young women known as *Filles de Charité* were brought in to assist the society. When St. Vincent sent Mlle. Le Gras to inspect his societies throughout the provinces, she decided that these *Filles* were everywhere needed and should receive some preparation for their work. She thereupon took groups of them into her own home for this purpose. Here St. Vincent gave them a series of talks on nursing ideals, and simple regulations were provided. Subsequent to such general training, the *Filles* were sent out to the provinces. Usually the *Dames de Charité*, who made up the local societies, would employ one of them to serve as a visiting lay nurse in their particular parish. Following the interests of St. Vincent, these young women gave particular attention to foundlings.

Although originally concerned with home nursing, the *Dames* soon realized that they and their *Filles* could also be well employed in hospitals. A society was formed in Paris, with the approval of the Archbishop, to assist in the Hôtel-Dieu. Here St. Vincent directed them to cooperate with the Augustinian Sisters who continued in charge of the halls, and the new lay helpers were accepted for supplementary employments without any friction. In 1639 some of the *Filles* were requested to take over the nursing in a hospital at Angers. They were provided with board and lodging by the hospital and were in turn subject to its regulations concerning the patients.

In 1642 the *Filles* began to take annual vows and assumed the title of Sister but were not to be viewed as "religious." St. Vincent de Paul opposed their forming a regular order in the traditional manner, lest this interfere with their freedom in nursing. No doubt some of the Sisters themselves may have desired the cloister because of the dignity or protection it afforded. At least this is implied in the famous statement of the founder, in which he declared: "My daughters, you are not nuns; and if any wrong-headed person appeared among you who should say, 'We ought to be nuns—that would be a much finer thing,' Ah, my daughters, the company would be at its last gasp . . . for whoever says the word *nun* says *cloister,* and the Sisters should go about everywhere."[34] By taking only annual vows, some degree of professional freedom was maintained. At the same time the scattered individuals or local groups throughout France were brought together in a somewhat stronger organization, under Mlle. Le Gras as Superior.

Between 1645 and 1660 the home visitations of the Sisters of Charity were continued, but they also took over the nursing in one French hospital after another. In each case they agreed to follow the regulations of these institutions, but in religious and disciplinary matters remained under the direction of their motherhouse. Some of the places in which they served were general hospitals; others were devoted to the care of such special groups as old workmen or the insane. In 1654 they began nursing wounded French soldiers, which is interesting in view of the usual attitude in Latin countries concerning the care of men. Indeed, in this respect they were far in advance of common practice in English-speaking countries, where only orderlies were provided in military hospitals down to the middle of the nine-

[34] Quoted in A. M. Lovat, *Life of the Venerable Louise de Marillac* (Mlle Le Gras), (London, 1916), 376, 377.

teenth century. The appeal which aroused Florence Nightingale in 1854 was a letter sent from the Crimean front, concluding with the dramatic question: "Why have we no Sisters of Charity?"

Mlle. Le Gras proved an able superior. She kept in personal touch with her Sisters throughout France and, as their activities spread, in countries as distant as Poland. Over seven hundred of her letters have been preserved. In them it is evident that she was zealously striving to provide a more effective system of nursing for both hospitals and homes in France. When she died in 1660 there were about 350 of her Sisters serving in some seventy institutions, and their work was expanded during the next two centuries.

It would seem as if the Sisters of Charity achieved all that a nursing group could do, given the religious ideal but as yet denied scientific enlightenment. The ordinary medical practice of 1650 was such that there was no point in establishing schools of nursing in hospitals. Nor was there as yet any appreciation of a truly medical role for nurses. Nursing reformers could not take this step until such an appreciation appeared and until there was sufficient science in nursing to make a technical training seem desirable.

While new nursing orders were being developed during the 1600's, both Church and State in Catholic Europe continued their efforts to adjust hospitals to changing times. The Council of Trent provided plans for reorganizing those which remained under clerical control. Wherever possible, these were placed under diocesan direction, and bishops were directed to visit them and to enforce proper procedures. All officials were to be held responsible to the episcopal authorities and were subject to censure or removal. If necessary, even the endowments could be redistributed. St. Charles Borromeo, who as a papal secretary was active at Trent, founded a hospital at Milan as an example of the Council's ideal. This is said to have been one of the first institutions in which the directors were required to submit reports at regular intervals.

This program for improved supervision seems to have been followed in most Catholic countries. Wherever nationalistic feeling and State power reached a certain stage, however, the decisions of councils as well as of popes were likely to be resisted or ignored. In Austria, for example, the larger hospitals came under the direction of royal authority, and eventually it was the Emperor there who directed attempted reforms. But the injection of State control was most marked in France, where secular trends were more advanced than in southern Europe.

It was noted above that Charles IX, in 1561, had placed the small establishments under civil direction. His successors Louis XIII and Louis XIV went much further with governmental reorganization during the seventeenth century. Apparently convinced that lay control had not succeeded in making the many local hospitals efficient, most of these were closed by royal order. Between fifteen and sixteen hundred were thus suppressed. Their endowments were merged with those of larger institutions in the cities, and to these the villages were authorized to send a certain number of their sick poor. It is to be remembered that village foundations still followed the medieval tradition of providing general poor relief, and it doubtless seemed more efficient to send their sick to the real hospitals in the towns. At the same time the crown established new general hospitals in the cities, notably in Paris.

In effect, this closing of small relief institutions throughout France was similar to the suppression of the same type in England during the Reformation. It led, as in England, to a transition period when there was much suffering among the village poor. During the 1700's, under Louis XV and Louis XVI, the national government required villages to set up new, civil relief organizations corresponding to the British poor law boards. Again the same trends are to be observed in Catholic France as in Protestant England; namely, the substitution of civil in the place of ecclesiastic poor relief in the villages, and the separation of general relief from strictly hospital activities.

The whole process can be defended on the ground that civil relief was more systematic. Uniform provisions were made by the government in each locality, whereas church facilities had varied with the different endowments inherited from the Middle Ages. Hospital specialization in the care of the sick also presumably made for greater efficiency. Like the English, however, the French reorganization can be criticized because of the suffering of the transition period and also because of the relatively cold-blooded character of the civil, public charity which ensued.

Certain differences did appear in the French experience as compared with the English. Local French endowments were not seized by the Crown but were reserved for the poor by being transferred to the city hospitals. Considerable litigation followed, whereas in England the local establishments were closed outright and no legal protests were allowed. In France, the local religious orders were absorbed in other Church activities, whereas in England they were usually forced back into secular life. But the experience of both countries clearly foreshadowed modern trends towards state control and hospital specialization—trends which were only partly modified by the religious traditions of the nation concerned.

Development of Hospitals and Nursing in America

Of interest to Americans is the fact that the sixteenth and seventeenth centuries witnessed the planting of the first European colonies on this Continent, and the period therefore brought the first contacts between whites and Indians. The latter had their own folk and magic medicine, as suggested in the first chapter, and early settlers were often impressed by the native "medicine men." As a matter of fact, ordinary European practice—with its bleeding, sweating, and repulsive drugs—was as yet hardly on a higher plane than was that of the Indians. Colonists actually could learn things of value from these so-called primitives, notably of American medicinal plants such as cascara and cinchona bark.

It is a rather dramatic picture, this meeting of sophisticated Europeans with native peoples who knew nothing of medical science but who could nevertheless care for their sick almost as well as could the newcomers. But the first Spanish and French colonists had at least one advantage over the "red men." Because of their medieval Christian heritage, the former were familiar with hospitals and nursing Sisters, and they naturally transplanted these along with the rest of their culture to the New World. Even the civilized Indians of Mexico and of Peru had developed nothing in the way of such institutions. So advanced a people as the Mayas had possessed a remarkable architecture of temples and pyramids, some knowledge of mathematics and astronomy, and much lore about plants and drugs. But of hospitals and nurses there was no evidence.

During the 1500's Spain, following Columbus' voyages, rapidly established colonies from Mexico to Peru. Nearly a century before the first permanent settlements of other Europeans were made, this Spanish Empire became a large and energetic realm. Where the native peoples were of an advanced type, they survived to mingle their blood and culture with that of the conquerors. But in the chief centers, as in Lima and Mexico City, Spanish civilization was established much as it was in the homeland. The medical science of the Renaissance was cultivated in the universities founded in these two cities (1550). And in them were built the first hospitals on this side of the Atlantic. No study of their operation is available, but they resembled Spanish hospitals at home in being served by nursing orders.

The first permanent settlements of the French and of the English were made about 1607. The contrast between them, in regard to hospitals and nursing, is rather striking. The French, like the Spaniards, naturally introduced these institutions in their chief colonial towns as soon as was feasible. The first hospital in Canada was the Hôtel-Dieu in Montreal (1655). This was the very period when Mlle. de Le Gras was organizing the Sisters of Charity in France; and it is not surprising that the pioneer Canadian hospital was also established by a devoted lay woman—Mademoiselle Jeanne Mance. Three Sisters of one of the smaller nursing orders assisted her there in caring for sick settlers and Indians.

A few years before this, several Augustinian Sisters sailed from France to Quebec, where they eventually (1658) were able to establish the Hôtel-Dieu of that city. Both here and at Montreal, the Sisters found their little hospitals all too inadequate for the desperate needs of pioneer communities. Certain fevers, especially malaria, typhoid, and dysentery, always flared up in the settlements. The colonists were often puzzled as to why the first years in a new site were usually healthy ones, only to be followed by "a great sickness." This can now be understood in terms of the infection of the local mosquito populations with malarial parasites, and by the gradual pollution of water supplies.

In addition to the sick, the Sisters had to look after other unfortunates. There were at first no special homes or asylums of any sort. In a word, frontier conditions were similar to those which had existed in northern Europe in the early Middle Ages, when the first Christian hospitals had been all things to all men. So the first French hospitals in America reverted to this primitive form, in which the sick,

171

the orphans, and the aged were all cared for under the same roof. One can observe the same arrangements, during the next century, in the well-known Charity Hospital of New Orleans.

The English settlers along the Atlantic Seaboard did not benefit from such institutions even in their larger towns. Since the English colonists came over nearly a century after the Reformation, they took it for granted that welfare work was a function of private charity or of the State. It does not seem to have occurred to English denominations, like the "Puritans" (Congregationalists) of New England, or the Anglicans (Episcopalians) in the Southern Colonies, that their churches might establish hospitals or asylums of any kind.

In any case, most of the people lived in thinly settled areas where it would have been difficult to provide such establishments. Nor did this sparsity of population permit a system of local "poor law boards" such as had already been established in Elizabethan England. In southern New England, where small towns were the rule, it was assumed that families could look after their own unfortunates and that "poor houses" were therefore unnecessary. In cases of extreme poverty, and the sickness which often accompanied this, the town authorities gave "outdoor relief"—providing small funds or boarding paupers out with other families. But this was done only for established residents. Any sick stranger who drifted into a village was viewed as a threat to the civic treasury, and he was hustled out of town much as tramps were in later years. Times had changed since the days when medieval hostels were open to all comers.

When English Colonial towns reached a certain size, however, some sort of public refuge had to be provided. Boston established an almshouse about 1680, similar to those set up earlier in English cities; and Philadelphia took similar action about 1730. (Each of these communities had existed for some fifty years before this step was finally forced upon it.) Since these almshouses provided infirmaries for sick inmates, they are sometimes viewed as the first hospitals in the English Colonies. This interpretation is plausible in those cases, such as that of Philadelphia, where the asylum infirmary later evolved into a municipal hospital.

Yet the mere existence of an infirmary in an almshouse did not make it a hospital in the modern sense. The sick received only casual medical attention, and such nursing as they secured was just provided by the other paupers. Enlightened citizens in the chief cities therefore urged the founding of real hospitals after the English model. Finally, about 1750, Dr. Thomas Bond and other Philadelphia physicians proposed that a general hospital be established there and sought contributions to make this possible. Aided by Benjamin Franklin, they secured funds from the Province (State) of Pennsylvania as well as from private donors; and the Pennsylvania Hospital was thus founded as the first institution of its kind in the English Colonies.

The original building of this Hospital is still in use and well illustrates the best hospital architecture of the eighteenth century. Although it received State aid when founded, the Pennsylvania Hospital was controlled by a private board just as were its counterparts in London. It was therefore a "voluntary" institution of the English type, and the first hospitals subsequently founded in other American cities followed this model. Only later did municipal (government) hospitals evolve from the almshouses, as noted above.

Both voluntary and municipal hospitals provided free care to the poor, and the municipal hospitals dealt only with this class. But voluntary institutions in this country also took in a few paying patients and even provided private rooms for them. In this respect, the American voluntary institutions differed from the English, since the latter—as is true of municipal institutions in America—served no private patients. The introduction of private care in a place like the Pennsylvania Hospital probably made for good standards of operation, since the well-to-do patronized it and were concerned about its reputation. In America, as in England, no trained nurses were available; but one did not hear such complaints about the nursing services in Philadelphia as one did in London.

The provision of private service in American institutions also suggested a new idea; namely, that prosperous patients might sometimes secure better treatment in a hospital than was available even in good homes. This idea would not fully develop for another century, when scientific advances would make hospital care mandatory for many cases. When this time came, American hospitals were already accustomed to having private patients and simply had to expand their facilities. The English, in contrast, were too class-conscious to send private patients to hospitals associated only with charity; and so they evolved small, separate institutions ("nursing homes") to take care of the upper social levels. But all this belongs to the later story.

Chapter IX

Science and Society in the
Eighteenth Century

The eighteenth century, prior to the American Revolution, has sometimes been considered a rather dull period. The greatest days of discovery and exploration were past; the dramatic religious wars were over; the sudden brilliance of the new science either died down or else men became more accustomed to its rays. It is easy to say, for example, that England in 1750 was a dull place in comparison with the brave days of Elizabeth or with the surging times of Cromwell and the civil wars. In like manner Louis XV of France could not maintain the glories of Louis XIV (the "grand monarch"); nor the rulers of decadent Spain, the somber grandeur of Philip II. And everyone knew that Italy, deprived of its once rich oriental trade by the Atlantic seaboard nations, was slipping from both commercial and cultural preeminence.

All of these developments, however, may be looked upon in another way. It was really fortunate that the religious wars ended about 1650; and that, despite smoldering antagonisms, Catholics and Protestants could go about their business without recurrent conflicts. There were wars enough between rival states, without adding those due to religious differences. It was just as well, too, that a period of early European expansion was followed by a steady development of colonies and trade; for this meant that Europe could "cash in" on early geographical gambles and so cultivate both its material and cultural concerns.

Much the same thing may be said of American developments. The English colonies of 1750 were not the exciting places that they had been a century or so before. The settlement of Georgia about 1730 was a prosaic matter compared with the struggle for survival at Jamestown in 1607, or at Plymouth in 1620. But the colonies were well established and making progress by the mid-eighteenth century; whereas the dramatic pioneer settlements of Captain John Smith and of Governor Bradford had seemed for a time little more than forlorn hopes. Hostile Indians had been picturesque, no doubt, but white men were thankful that the natives had by this time been removed to another world or at least to the other side of the mountains.

In other words, the first half of the eighteenth century seems a bit stuffy because it was not a pioneering period. It was rather a time between major conflicts, when Europe and America were temporarily able to settle down and to develop the wealth and ideas which had been inherited from preceding years. And it is in just such periods that substantial progress is often made. It was unfortunate but perhaps inevitable that this led in turn to new difficulties, that religious tensions were replaced by class and national conflicts. And those who like their history in dramatic form may be reconciled to the eighteenth century by its final years, when it witnessed the advent of industrialism and came to a close amidst the frantic upheavals of the French Revolution.

Industrial and Economic Developments—The Industrial Revolution

The economic developments of the 1700's were most important but can be only summarized here. Agriculture continued to be the occupation of most Europeans, who labored as serfs on manorial estates or, in some cases, as free men on small holdings. Farming was a hard but fairly efficient occupation among peasants, who cultivated it as a folk art and a way of life. Only in England had these people, freed from serfdom, been driven in many cases to the towns because landlords preferred to enclose their estates and raise sheep for wool. English towns had therefore long been plagued with "sturdy beggars" (unemployed) who had forgotten how to farm and could find little to do in trade or handicrafts.

This was why so many Englishmen went to the American colonies; and why, once there, few of them proved to be really good farmers. They had little feel for the soil as did French or German peasants, and proceeded to exhaust it in an effort to "get rich quick" and so escape from the hard way of life to which true peasants were devoted. As long as land was plentiful and cheap, this careless cultivation paid well; but it established a habit of wasteful agriculture that was later to threaten parts of the United States with sheer ruin. Those who know the difficulties of modern "share croppers" will understand some of the later consequences of this unfortunate tradition.

Toward the end of the century, the spread of scientific ideas led to attempts to apply science to farming as well as to navigation, manufacturing and other arts. Improvements were made in farm implements, as in making plows of iron rather than of wood; the rotation of crops was studied in order to increase soil fertility; and better breeding produced more valuable livestock. As a result, our present breeds of sheep and cattle are almost twice as large as were medieval stocks. Much of this early "scientific agriculture" was the work of English gentlemen; but it came too late to keep the mass of English folk on the farms. It was little heeded at first in America, because land here was so cheap that it hardly paid to farm carefully. Eventually, however, the so-called agricultural revolution did better the methods employed all over the Western World, and this in turn improved the food supply of all but the poorest classes.

The steady increase in wealth after 1700 owed as much to trade and handicrafts as it did to agriculture. This, again, was quite marked in England. In the struggle for expanding trade with America and the East, England was most successful. In a series of wars with commercial rivals, she defeated Spain in 1583, Holland about 1660, and France in 1763. Through naval supremacy, Great Britain acquired most of North America, India, and other Oriental territories, and her trade became the greatest in the world. Only France survived as a major rival, although the overseas commerce of Spain, Portugal, and Holland remained substantial.

Leaders in all these competing countries agreed on one thing. They held that colonies existed in order to supply the mother-country with raw materials (wheat, tobacco, coffee) and to buy in return manufactured goods which the shops of the mother land could produce. The latter made money on such commerce both ways, and viewed its colonies as so many business agencies for its own advantage. This "mercantilist theory" worked well until the colonies decided they might do their own manufacturing or become independent in other ways, and then there was trouble.

If a colony were inhabited by divided peoples who lacked European weapons, as in India, it could be controlled; but if it were occupied by men of European descent who shared the ambitions of the mother country, this was not so easy. When Great Britain decided to "tighten up" on the American Colonies after 1765, in order to make them obey laws about trade and manufacturing, the Americans rebelled and achieved independence as the United States of America. About fifty years later, similar revolutions spread throughout the Spanish colonies and led to the creation of most of the present states of Latin America.

The desire of European merchants to sell their own products to America and to the Orient, naturally stimulated manufacturing at home. In 1700 goods were made either by workers in their own homes, or in the shops of master-workmen such as carpenters. These hand-made materials were usually of good quality and craftsmen took pride in their products. But the work was necessarily slow and the output small. What merchants needed was a quicker and cheaper way of turning out goods for sale, and the only solution of this problem was to improve the methods of production. Could better tools and processes be found?

The two most constant needs of any consuming public were food and clothing. No machines for the manufacture of the first were available in this period except the mills for grinding grain. But hand spinning wheels and looms had long been employed in preparing cloth for clothing and other purposes. Practical men began seeking improvements in these, to speed up the process and to give the merchants more cloth to sell. To make a long story short, first a device for spinning thread faster was invented and this piled up thread beyond the amount that the slow hand-loom could use. This led to the invention of a better loom which could weave more rapidly. That in turn could outdistance the supply of thread, and forced a second improvement of the spinning machines. So the process of invention shuttled back and forth through the 1700's.

Most of these improvements were made in England, partly because it had long been a weaving center but also for other reasons to be noted shortly. The new machines could be used for spinning various textiles—wool, linen, silk, and cotton. Wool and linen were plentiful in the British Isles; and after the invention of the cotton gin in Savannah about 1800, there was likewise a plentiful supply of American cotton.

Textile machines continued, at first, to be operated in homes. But as wheels and looms were made larger, they became too heavy for hand operation. They were then attached to big water wheels and this forced the workers to leave their homes and go to work in the mills. The only difficulty with this was that a textile mill had to be located on a stream giving water power. If some other form of power could be used, location could be made independent of this factor. This need, as well as other possible uses, stimulated inventors to improve the steam engines which had been used for pumping water since about 1690.

As a result, steam engines capable of operating whole rows of textile machines were developed before the end of the century. Such a setup, even more than that of a water mill, required the location of many machines in a special building known as a factory. And as factories multiplied, manufacturing ceased to be a hand process in homes and became more and more a matter of machine production in large-scale establishments. This was true not only in the output of textiles, but also in the development of iron mills for the making of all kinds of machinery and other metal products.

The early "industrial revolution" occurred first in England (1750–1800). Here there was the old weaving tradition, and here also were available the coal and iron needed for making and operating machinery. The English had other advantages as well. They had accumulated wealth from earlier trade expansion and so had the funds required for building factories and setting up new businesses. Just because of earlier trade, moreover, merchants were an influential class in England and the Government tended to favor business interests in general.

For one thing, the British Government did all it could to foster commerce both at home and abroad. Since the new factories could produce more textiles and tools than ever before, efforts had to be made to sell ever larger amounts of goods. This meant, among other things, a demand for better transportation between factories and markets. British roads were improved and stagecoach lines established, while port facilities were improved and shipping expanded. Inventors even began to put steam engines in land and water vehicles in order to speed up travel. Hence, by 1800, the transportation system in England—as well as its mines and factories—foreshadowed an industrial era.

Evils and Benefits Resulting from the Industrial Revolution

The advent of the steam engine was a turning point in history. Up to this time, men had first used their own hands in making and transporting goods, then had employed animals, and had finally enlisted the power of wind and water. But steam was a new type of power—the first that men could make themselves when and where they needed it. Combined with new machines, steam could produce more and cheaper articles for human use than had ever before been available. It therefore promised to improve man's standard of living wherever it was employed.

Actually, however, the story was not quite so simple as that. In some ways, the industrial revolution—powered by steam—did bring many benefits; but in other respects the results seemed harmful. Since all this happened first in England, the results were first observable there, but many of them were repeated later whenever manufacturing was introduced in other countries.

Most obvious among the benefits were those secured by the business classes. Fortunes were made and such people began to live more comfortably than ever before. National wealth also mounted and increased funds became available for art, education and science. Although these things were chiefly enjoyed by the upper classes, even the masses benefited when transportation improved, food became more plentiful, and clothing cheaper.

The fact that cotton garments were easily washable, for example, encouraged cleanliness; which in turn gave some protection against filth diseases. So, too, did the manufacture of iron bedsteads which— unlike the old wooden ones—were not liable to infestation with vermin. Such improvements in living conditions were not planned as health measures; they were just by-products of manufacturing which happened to have health values.

At the same time, a conscious demand arose for advancing public welfare. Just because the upper classes were enjoying higher standards than ever before, their more conscientious leaders became aware of contrasts in the condition of the poor. Could not something be done to provide the masses with at least some of the benefits which greater wealth had already brought to the more fortunate classes?

As soon as philanthropists began looking into the condition of the poor, they often found that things were worse than had been realized. Traditional charity evidently was not enough; systematic efforts must be made to remedy social evils. This had to be done not only out of sympathy, but also because bad living conditions weakened the nation. If workers were ill, for example, industry suffered as well as the people themselves. A national interest in social reform was thus added to the old impulses of Christian benevolence.

Out of this state of mind arose various reform movements which would go on into the next century; for example, the temperance and the antislavery crusades. Of particular interest here were the efforts made to improve the health of the masses. The poor obviously suffered more from disease than did the comfortable classes, and this was apparently a result of poor living conditions and hygiene. The living conditions could not be immediately improved, as will be noted shortly; but something might be done to promote better hygiene through education.

Some vital statistics were becoming available by the 1700's, and these indicated that the highest death rates were those among infants. Certain physicians and others therefore embarked on a campaign for improving the care of babies. They opened dispensaries for mothers and wrote pamphlets on infant care—urging proper clothing, food, and nursing. They had to overcome all sorts of folk lore about swaddling clothes, feeding pork to the newborn in order to "cure them of their mother's longings," and so on. The reformers also urged physicians to see the babies and not to leave them to the care of "old women." (Practitioners had heretofore done little for infants, since such patients were unable to describe symptoms.) Here was the beginning of a conscious concern about pediatrics.

Between 1750 and 1800, the infant death rate in England began to fall for the first time, and this trend can be ascribed in part to the infant welfare movement. The average infant mortality, 1731–1740, had been appalling—about 437 deaths per 1,000 births—but by 1791–1800 this figure had fallen to 240.[35] Here was a gain of almost 50 per cent in fifty years!

The decrease in infant deaths was bound to affect the crude death rate of the entire English nation. This is estimated to have been about 36 per 1,000 in 1731–1740; but by 1791–1800 had declined to about 27. Other evidence indicates that the improvement resulted almost entirely from the saving of life during the first year. Since the birth rate continued high, meantime, the fall in crude mortality inevitably led to an increase in total population.

Such an increase was to follow in all Western countries during the next century, after the industrial revolution set in, and is one of the most striking phenomena of modern history. If carried too far, it may threaten a country with over-population; and as early as about 1800, the British scientist Malthus was viewing the growth of his nation's numbers with alarm. Some critics even advised against efforts to improve the people's health, lest these preserve too many mouths to feed. Yet, at the time, population growth in England could be viewed as a sign of better conditions among the masses.

All this, however, is but one side of the story—the favorable side of industrialization and the reform movements which came with it. More attention has often been given to the unhappy aspects of the picture. As manufacturing expanded in England, it became concentrated in factory towns. And into these poured the workers from villages and country-side, to live in crowded slums around the mills. Women and children were employed because their wages were lower than those of men, and the work was long (12 to 16 hours were not uncommon) and monotonous. Overworked and underpaid, denied decent housing, food and recreation, the workers often found their only escape in drink and became easy victims of tuberculosis and other fevers.

How much worse off these people were in the mill towns than they had been in villages, is impossible to say. Certain it is that, while the total population of England was rising by 1800, the rate of in-

[35] By 1945, in the United States, this figure (deaths under 1 year, per 1,000 births) was about 38.

crease in its large cities was below the average. Deaths were so high in London that the population there would have declined, had not people kept coming in. And, in any case, human misery was certainly concentrated and made more obvious in the urban slums than it had ever been in rural surroundings.

The industrial revolution thus brought evils as well as benefits to society. In time, the sufferings of the laboring class in England—and elsewhere—would bring further efforts at reform. Before one considers this later, nineteenth-century story, however, it were well to recall the social changes which occurred during the 1700's in other lands besides Great Britain.

Developments in Politics, Science and Women's Rights

In 1800 only the British possessed manufacturing facilities and "know-how." They "got the jump" on other countries, and British trade and wealth surpassed that of any other land. Although the spread of the factory system to other lands was almost inevitable, the process was delayed elsewhere by various factors.

In the small cities of the United States, for example, merchants rarely had enough funds (capital) to build factories before about 1830. And even in Continental Europe, no such mercantile wealth had accumulated as in England. It happened, also, that certain old areas such as Italy lacked coal and iron. In others, society was still dominated by monarchs and nobles who had little interest in "vulgar" trade, and who were content with keeping life just as it had always been.

The latter situation was best illustrated in the case of France. Although French commerce had increased in the 1600's, merchants and the middle classes remained somewhat subservient to the landed aristocrats. Ambitious kings maintained glittering courts and wasted funds in efforts to enlarge the kingdom. There were wars and glory, but the burden of all this fell on hard-working peasants and over-taxed businessmen. For these and other reasons, the factory system was not introduced in France during the 1700's. Instead of growing in power, the French middle class felt handicapped and thwarted, and resentment was built up which threatened political as well as economic repercussions.

Louis XVI completed the bankruptcy of his government when he sent fleets and armies to America to help the patriots there win their independence in 1783. Then he had to turn to the middle classes for financial aid and the latter began to take things into their own hands. In the French Revolution which followed, the old order was overturned and society was changed even more than it had been in England. The peasants seized the estates of the landlords and the titled aristocracy was abolished. Guilds were destroyed and free business competition substituted. Manufacturing was encouraged and outworn traditions like cruel punishments were eliminated.

The French, as noted, went further than the British. Something should be done for farmers, for workers, and for other poor folk. All men should have the right to vote. There should be no privileged institutions. Even the Church was attacked, since its wealth and connection with the nobility made it appear aristocratic to the revolutionists. Its property was confiscated and placed in the hands of the State. Contemplative religious orders were abolished, but those devoted to nursing and other forms of social service were permitted to remain. Radical leaders, influenced by skeptical thought which had grown out of science after 1750, finally advocated the suppression of all religion. A woman dressed as the "Goddess of Reason" was worshiped in mock ceremony on the high altar of Notre Dame in Paris.

The Paris mob, bitter against the upper classes, supported these extremes and executed all who opposed them. The resulting "Reign of Terror" was too much for the middle classes. They began to realize that, having eliminated the nobility who had been above them in the social scale, they were now threatened by the masses who were below them. Here was foreshadowed that conflict between the middle and working classes, between capital and labor, which was to become so serious after 1850. Meanwhile the French middle classes turned to a strong leader, Napoleon Bonaparte, in an effort to bring order out of chaos.

Napoleon proved to be half revolutionary reformer, half reactionary dictator. He ruled France like an all-powerful monarch and tried to extend his Empire throughout Europe. Eventually he was overthrown by a coalition of European powers at the battle of Waterloo in 1815. But wherever his armies went in Europe they overthrew petty princes, abolished serfdom and guilds, and opened the way for middle-class business regimes. After his downfall, limited monarchies replaced the old absolute governments in France, Germany, and Italy, and the way was paved for both national unity and democratic reforms in those lands.

Most important here, Napoleon realized that expanding trade and industry were dependent on technology—on tools and machines—and that the latter in turn were influenced ultimately by science. He therefore encouraged scientific men and institutions in Paris and made that city the scientific capital of the world. Among other things, he reorganized the hospitals and medical schools, and this provided research opportunities that had much to do with revolutionizing medical science.

The leaders of the French Revolution felt that they were sweeping the last vestiges of medieval tradition from Europe. Serfdom, the guilds, and the titled aristocracy were all viewed as parts of the medieval inheritance. There was to be a new freedom—freedom for peasants to farm their own lands, for businessmen to develop trade and manufacturing, for all men to participate in government and to think as they chose. And not only "all men." Why not women as well?

If men deserved new liberties—the argument ran—the feminine half of the race stood in even greater need of liberation. For whatever restrictions were imposed upon a man in any class, his wife was still largely under *his* domination. She had little control over her own person, property, or children. Single women might have better legal status but had access to few opportunities above the level of domestic service or labor in the mills. For middle-class females, marriage remained the only vocation.

During the French Revolution, a delegation of women appealed to the National Assembly to extend the same rights to the one sex as to the other. This was denied at the time; but underlying economic and social changes were moving in that direction. In England the poorer women were working in the mills, and middle class matrons had secured a leisure which led them to ponder their position. Women's rights and wrongs began to be a matter of public debate in both Europe and America. In Philadelphia, for example, a magazine devoted to women's interests was established as early as the 1790's. Eventually, such activities would expand into a conscious feminist campaign—one of the many social reform movements of the time.

Revolt Against Things Medieval

The general revolt against things medieval, which was expressed dramatically in the French Revolution, influenced nearly all aspects of society and culture. It was a sort of second Renaissance, and reformers sought to remove those aspects of medievalism which had survived the first Renaissance. As once before in the 1500's, leaders of the 1700's looked back to classical times for inspiration. Although there had been no precedents in Greece or Rome for the newer developments of the eighteenth century, such as industrialism, philosophers could find classical models for many things.

In political life, for example, the new governments in both the United States and France set up Senates—because the Senate had been the governing body in early Rome. The study of Roman law was renewed and politicians imitated the oratory of Athenian masters. Even the feminist appeal might be viewed as a return to Roman viewpoints, which had permitted women a large degree of freedom in imperial days.

Education and the fine arts also were affected by the second classic revival. French and American senators had statues made of themselves clad in Roman togas. (You can still see them in the Capitol at Washington.) The dress of women in this "Empire period" took on the loose, flowing lines of classical costume. Schools assumed the Greek names of "academy" and "lyceum," and a learned society in the United States selected Greek letters (Phi Beta Kappa) for its name. Painters delighted in classical scenes, and architecture reverted to reproduction of Greco-Roman styles. Instead of late Renaissance forms like English Georgian and American "Colonial" (in which classical lines had been greatly modified), there was substituted the original Greek temple in all its austere dignity. The only change was that instead of using this type only for religious buildings, it was now employed for homes, banks, and other purposes. In their main buildings New York and Philadelphia began to look like Greek or Roman cities, somewhat as Washington does today on a grander scale.

Expansion of the Sciences

While the fine arts were thus returning to earlier forms, the sciences continued to go forward in terms of ever increasing knowledge. The fine arts expressed the culture of a given period but they rarely determined the basic nature of that culture. Science and technology, on the other hand, usually kept moving in one direction and actually changed the character of civilization from one epoch to the next. Thus the shift about 1800 from Renaissance art to "Greek Revival" reflected a change in taste but did not otherwise alter the character of European life in that era. But the transfer from wind machines to steam engines, or from hand looms to power looms at the same time, profoundly altered the whole way of life for millions of people.

The major changes which came in with the factory system resulted from practical inventions (technology or engineering), rather than from science proper. The man who invented a new machine or process was still, in most cases, ignorant of physics. But physicists did take some interest in steam engines, and they were the ones who would eventually find still other sources of power. The time would come when even practical inventions would be based on scientific knowledge, and this outcome was the result of scientific advances already under way before 1800.

Continued progress was made in the natural sciences during the eighteenth century, by virtue of the relatively new methods already established in the 1600's. Experimentation, measurements, and the use of instruments of observation were now taken for granted in certain fields. Many advances were made in physics, chemistry, and biology, but one need recall here only those which had some meaning for medicine.

In physics, interest shifted from the observation of moving bodies (dynamics) to a study of forms of energy—of light, heat, and electricity. In breaking white light into colors (as any prism will do, or as raindrops accomplish in the rainbow), physicists became interested in the reverse process. How, that is, could colored light be recombined into white? The problem was a practical one, since the lenses in telescopes or microscopes broke up white light into colors and this confused anyone who used them. In 1758 a London optician, cooperating with physicists in Holland and Sweden, invented an achromatic (noncolored) telescope which greatly aided astronomers. And finally, about 1830, lens makers in Paris, Berlin, and other centers succeeded in making similar achromatic microscopes. The value of these to medical scientists was obvious; without such improved instruments later work in cellular pathology and bacteriology would have been impossible. Other French scientists, studying the effect of light rays on "sensitive" plates covered with certain chemicals, discovered the process known as photography. This also was later of great use in medicine.

The study of heat was advanced after 1700 by the invention of better measuring instruments. Galileo had used a thermometer which simply measured the expansion of hot air in a glass tube. Later, mercury was used instead of air and could be measured more exactly. No one could at first agree on just what scale should be used in these instruments—as many as thirteen different ones were employed in 1740. Finally a Swedish scientist, Celsius, introduced in 1742 the centigrade scale which came into general use in scientific circles. The scale used by the German, G. D. Fahrenheit, now survives only in English-speaking lands. Although thermometers were rarely employed by doctors before 1850, they were subsequently found of great value in medical practice.

Research in electricity attracted increasing attention during the 1700's. Static electricity was studied in "Leyden jars," which could produce sparks and shocks which amused those who experienced them. Everyone remembers the experiment of the American, Benjamin Franklin, whose kite proved that lightning was just a huge spark of this sort. It is a wonder he was not injured; indeed, two Russians who repeated the experiment were killed. Franklin pointed out that the "electrical fire" might some day be used for practical purposes like cooking, and meanwhile he invented the lightning rod to protect men against its heavenly activities.

No such practical use for electricity in medicine appeared for some time. It is of interest, nevertheless, that the next great step in this field was the discovery of current electricity by an Italian anatomist, Galvani. This medical scientist observed a current passing through a muscle-nerve preparation when it was accidentally touched by a metal bar. Further study of electrical currents later made possible such important inventions as the telegraph and the dynamo. Thus, doctors not only benefited from physical science but themselves contributed to it.

Alchemists, with their mystical search for gold, were discredited after 1700. In their place appeared chemists who wished to discover natural laws about chemical phenomena. The most obvious chemical phenomenon was the process of burning, and for long it was held that fire was itself a substance. This was called phlogiston and it was said to escape from materials whenever they were burned. (Hence doctors spoke of anti-phlogistic treatments; that is, against heat.) But the French chemist, Lavoisier, showed that mercury or other metals burnt in air actually gained weight (by adding oxygen in becoming oxides); hence they clearly lost no fire-substance. Later, by weighing carefully the materials involved in combustion, he showed just how much mercury and how much oxygen was present in the oxide product. This opened the way to a study of the composition of chemical compounds. Those which could not be broken down into simpler substances were called elements; and, reviving an old Greek theory, these were said in turn to be made up of atoms.

Lavoisier made further discoveries which, although of no immediate value to medical practice, exerted a great influence on the whole field of physiology. After an English chemist, Joseph Priestley, had discovered oxygen, Lavoisier found that this element combined with charcoal (carbon) to form carbonic acid gas. He noted that air in which carbon had been burned lost oxygen but gained in carbonic acid—because the oxygen had been combined with carbon in producing that gas. Then he observed that air exhaled by an animal showed the same results; that is, after leaving the lungs it had lost oxygen but gained in carbonic acid. The chemist concluded that oxygen combined in the lungs with carbon from the blood, just as it did with ordinary charcoal when this was burned in a vessel. In other words, respiration involved a type of combustion.

Lavoisier also demonstrated that when burning charcoal and a breathing animal each gave off the same amount of carbonic acid, they produced likewise the same amount of heat. Clearly, it was the burning process which was responsible for the heat in the animal as well as in the flaming charcoal. Here was a final answer to the old problem of the source of body heat. This resulted, not from friction as some had supposed, but simply from the combustion involved in the process of respiration.

The general view of early iatrochemists, such as Paracelsus, was thus at last confirmed. Two physiologic functions, respiration and heat production, were shown to be chemical processes. Hence, out of

Lavoisier's weighings and measurements, was born the new discipline of physiologic chemistry. It is a pity that so brilliant a scientist should have been executed as an aristocrat!

After Lavoisier's death, other scientists continued to study the relationships of chemical materials to biologic processes. Here, again, the results were not of immediate use to physicians, although they might have been if the doctors had fully realized their significance. In England, for example, one Dr. Beddoes founded a Pneumatic Institute, where research was conducted on the effects exerted by new gases on the human body. Here young Dr. Humphry Davy experimented with nitrous oxide, and found that its inhalation produced temporary unconsciousness. As early as about 1800, he declared, "It may probably be used to advantage in surgical operations." Surgeons, unfortunately, did not take the hint at the time; but certain gases were destined to be employed as anesthetics in the not too distant future.

When one turns from chemistry to the general biology of this period, the story seems rather remote from medicine. Yet profound changes were taking place in the study of botany and zoology. There were few such professional biologists as now work in universities, but physicians and others devoted much time to identifying the many living forms found in both the Old World and the New.

By the later 1700's, so many thousands of these forms were known as to be confusing and some scheme of classifying them was badly needed. Linnaeus, a Swedish physician, then provided a classification system—in terms of class, genus, and species—which is still used today in a modified manner. Thus, animals were divided into vertebrates and invertebrates; the former into the several classes of fishes, amphibia, reptiles, birds, and mammals; and mammals, as an example, into such genuses as the rodents, canine (dog-like) and feline (cat-like). Each of the genuses, finally, was broken down into separate species; for instance, the feline into such species as lions, tigers, and domestic cats.

Plants or animals were said to belong to the same genus because they were somewhat similar to each other. But what *were* their mutual relationships? Why were house cats and tigers at once so alike and so different? Had they been separately created? Or had one evolved from the other—or both from a common ancestor—and if so, just how? Thus arose the classic problem of "the origin of species."

Lamarck, a French zoologist, offered a theory in order to explain the evolution (gradual change) of one species into another. This had occurred, he held, because of "the inheritance of acquired characteristics." He suggested, as an illustration of this, that ancestral forms of giraffes had had short necks but had constantly made these longer by stretching them up into trees. Then the lengthened necks had been inherited by offspring, which in turn stretched them still further. Result, after thousands of years of this, the glorified giraffe neck as we now know it. In other words, one species of animal had here evolved into another of quite different appearance. It was assumed that similar evolution had gone on throughout the "animal kingdom" for indefinite lengths of time, and that this explained all contrasts and relationships between different forms.

William C. Wells, an American physician who moved from Charleston to London about 1783, proposed a different explanation of biologic evolution. The "inheritance of acquired characteristics" had no place in his theory. Instead, Wells would have explained the evolution of long necks as follows.

Originally, most ancestral giraffes had had short necks, and this quality was inherent in their heredity and was passed on to all their descendants. But when such animals lived in an area where their best food was tree foliage, they were unable to reach the leaves and so most of them did not survive long enough to reproduce themselves. The short-necks therefore tended to die off. Meantime, a few who were unusual in having long necks ("sports," or mutations) were able to eat well and to leave descendants. Since the quality of long-neck was inherent in these animals' germ cells, all their descendants retained it. Hence, in due time, the long-necks became common, while the short-necks disappeared. Result, after many thousands of years, the present species of giraffe. This theory therefore explained evolution as a process resulting from "the survival of the fittest."

Lamarck, Wells, and other "evolutionists" were developing their ideas at the end of the eighteenth century, but they made no great impression at that time. Not until Charles Darwin presented Wells' view in a more convincing manner, some half-century later (1859), would the theory of biologic evolution be generally accepted in scientific circles. Yet the efforts made as early as about 1800, to explain these problems, indicated a realization that present animal forms can be understood only in relation to their history. The same notion was also applied to other matters; for example, to the "evolution" of social institutions like hospitals. To know something fully, one has to know "how it got that way."

Dissemination of Scientific Information

Quite apart from particular discoveries in science and their implications for medicine, scientific thought influenced the whole outlook of the eighteenth century. In the 1600's, science had been an interest of only a small number of "philosophers." Their work, although brilliant, had been little known even among the upper classes. But by the 1700's, the number of printed books and journals increased, and those relating to science reached a wider audience. Public lectures also began to be given on scientific subjects. Benjamin Franklin, a printer in Philadelphia, had his interest aroused in electricity by hearing an itinerant lecturer discourse on electric sparks.

Public attention resulted, in part, from pure curiosity or even from a desire for entertainment. Mild electric shocks, for example, could amuse any audience. But educated men also became aware that scientific discoveries might have useful results. In Franklin's case, again, his research on electricity soon led to the invention of a protective lightening rod. Many other applications of science were made during the 1700's; as when physicists constructed thermometers and astronomers improved the art of navigation. Such things were obviously desirable, even as were the new machines produced by practical inventors. Science, combined with technology, thus came to promise much for the future of mankind.

If science had already accomplished so much, what limits could be set on its achievements in the future? True, its benefits might be selfishly reserved for the privileged few, but this thought was countered by the current desire for social reform. Why should not scientific advances go hand in hand with social amelioration? Perhaps science would even find means for overcoming poverty and disease and so point the way to utopia. The French thinker Condorcet, for example, predicted that medicine would eventually prevent or cure all diseases and so enable men to live on indefinitely.

These two ideas—that knowledge would ever grow, and then be applied increasingly to human welfare—were merged into a vision of "progress." (Both inventions, on the one hand, and social advances on the other, are still viewed as "signs of progress.") If men would only adopt a scientific attitude toward all problems—if they would control their prejudices and think clearly—the world could be made a better and better place for mankind. All that was needed to bring this about was time and "enlightenment."

Such a faith in progress is often said, today, to have been naive and over-optimistic. Wars and other tragedies have brought disillusionment to the present generation, which realizes that science can destroy as well as save. But in 1775 or 1800 there was much evidence in support of optimism; and meanwhile, this outlook provided an incentive for increased efforts in science and in social reform. Those who believed in progress had a goal which beckoned them on; their certainty of ultimate betterment made all their efforts seem worth while.

There was no area in which enlightenment was more needed than in medicine. Here was a field which combined science and social welfare in a peculiarly intimate manner, and it was no accident that philosophers—from Descartes to Condorcet—viewed its possibilities as central to the idea of progress.[36] But possibilities were one thing, the actual state of affairs quite another. In most respects, medical science seemed during the 1700's to lag behind the physical sciences.

This situation elicited questions and protests. Why was medicine not advancing in step with physics, chemistry, and technology? And what could be done about it? Such queries placed physicians on the defensive, and led some to say by 1800 that medicine must be completely made over in the likeness of physical science. So the idea of progress did have an impact on medicine—even if in a negative sort of way—and this will be the theme of the ensuing chapter.

[36] Descartes had declared that: *"Si l'espèce humaine peut être perfectionée, c'est dans la médecine qu'il faut en chercher les moyens."*

Chapter X

Medicine Gropes for Light:

1700 to 1800

During the eighteenth century medical developments were by no means as clear as were those in physical science or general biology. The theories of physicians now seem to have been confused, and their practice static or even reactionary. At the same time, technical advances continued in certain medical arts, contributions were made by folk medicine, and the training and institutions available to medical men were improved. Looking back, one may say that medicine was groping in the dark but was seeking light with growing anticipation. New concepts as well as further knowledge were essential if light was to be found.

Consider, first, the trends in the traditional medical sciences—in anatomy, physiology, and pathology.[37] Advances made in normal, gross anatomy during the 1700's were not striking, since the basic knowledge had already been acquired. More careful research was done on particular organs, such as the teeth and the nervous system, and interesting comparisons were undertaken between the structures of man and of other animals (comparative anatomy). But there were no major discoveries in normal anatomy such as those earlier achieved by Vesalius.

---

[37] Traditionally, these were the essential medical sciences, while therapy, surgery, and hygiene were more arts than sciences. Logically, however, one may think of pathology and therapy as central to medicine, in which case anatomy and physiology can be viewed simply as branches of biology basic to medicine.

Similar comments may be made on the history of physiology during this era. Earlier research had shown that physical methods could be used in this field with brilliant results. In demonstrating the circulation of blood, for example, Harvey had used measurements (quantitative method) and experiments; and Malphigi had employed the microscope. Experimental studies were continued when, about 1750, the Swiss physician Albrecht von Haller investigated the nervous system. He was able, by using animals, to distinguish between motor and sensory responses. Crude attempts were also made to reveal the chemistry of digestion; and toward the end of the century, Lavoisier made his great discoveries concerning respiration and body heat. Clearly, we would now say, physiology could be best advanced if its complexities could be reduced to the terms of physical science.

During the eighteenth century, however, the situation did not appear as simple as this. In the first place, it was not easy to select the most significant problems presented by the behavior of the human body. Should medical scientists focus on normal processes or on spectacular abnormalities—on further studies of circulation or on the latest village monstrosity? Moreover, when attention was centered on basic processes—on circulation, digestion, or nervous action—the application of physical methods then available was often unsuccessful.

Measurements, for example, brought different results with different men. When attempts were made to measure the force of the heart pump, one physician reported this to be a matter of fifty pounds, another found it to be only one. Again, what observer "A" saw under the microscope could not always be confirmed by observers "B" and "C." Such discrepancies were confusing; and led to the conclusion that life processes, in their very nature, were too complex for measurement or analysis.

Many scientists went further in deciding that organisms could never be fully understood in terms of physics and chemistry. There must be some "vital principle" inherent in all living forms—including the human body—which made them behave differently from inanimate things. And how could one measure or experiment with anything so vague as a vital principle?

Partly because of this viewpoint, few medical men made serious studies in physiology. Most of them were physicians who, as mentioned before, could see little value in laboratory research as far as their practice was concerned. The experienced physician, they held, could develop an intuitive sense for a patient's condition and needs; and was this not more essential than to dabble with instruments and experiments? Scientists might well measure physical materials, but the human body was too complex—and the human mind too subtle—for this sort of thing.

So widespread was this view that practitioners did not even employ such simple measurements as might have been used in everyday practice. By 1600, Italian scientists had invented air thermometers for taking body temperature; yet clinical thermometers did not come into common use until after 1850. Nor were watches used to time the pulse until that later era, although a pulse-watch was invented as early as 1730. Learned physicians considered it beneath their dignity to employ such artificial contrivances.

Varied Interpretations of Developments in Medical Science

One of the instruments which was largely neglected after 1700 was the microscope. Most observers could not use it as well as did Leeuwenhoek, the inventor, and the latter trained no students to continue his work. More than a century later an American, Oliver Wendell Holmes, referred to microscopy as "an art now almost forsaken." Such indifference had unfortunate results. Had this instrument been improved more rapidly and used more intensively, it would have revealed a new world in anatomy—that of microscopic structure or histology. But only occasional attempts were made along this line until well after 1830.

It is true that microscopy had introduced a novel idea into pathology as early as the 1600's—Kircher's concept of microorganisms as the causes of infection. During the early 1700's, there was widespread interest in this "germ theory." Some physicians supported it by the evidence of disease behavior (epidemiology); as when they argued that "consumption" acted as if it were caused and spread by minute "insects" or "worms." But simple observation of this sort was not enough; microscopic studies and experiments were needed to prove or disprove the hypothesis. And here there were difficulties, of both a technical and conceptual nature, which were not overcome until long after 1800.

First, the microscopes of the period were relatively crude and

197

ineffective ones. Nor was there any awareness of the need for staining "germs," if they were to be well seen. Equally serious was the fact that physicians could not even look for the causal factors in any malady, until they knew just what this form of illness was and how to recognize it. And the pathology of the 1700's—the third medical science mentioned above—was still unable to identify many disease entities. Imagine searching for the bacteria involved in so vague a condition as "griping of the guts," when no one knew the difference between typhoid, dysentery, and other types of gastrointestinal infections.

Here one should recall what has already been said about the pathology of preceding centuries. This science of the nature and causes of disease was obviously central to all medical thought and practice. Most physicians of the 1700's continued to accept the old pathologic theory that all disease—regardless of particular symptoms —resulted from some one, underlying condition that involved the body as a whole. (We still employ such generalized concepts when we speak of "being in bad condition" or of "being all run down.") Most common was the old view that illness resulted from the state of the blood or other fluids, and that treatment therefore should relieve the body of fluids through bleeding, purging, and sweating.

All physicians knew a number of different symptom patterns which led them, for example, to speak of smallpox as being something different from chickenpox or measles. But if all three of these resulted from the general state of the blood, distinctions between them were not important—one bled or purged in any case.

A divergent view had been held by Sydenham in the 1600's, however, when he insisted that these and other symptom patterns revealed entirely different diseases—each of which had its own particular cause and required particular means for prevention or cure. If so, the great problem in pathology was to identify as many different diseases as possible. "Instead of theorizing about disease in general," said Sydenham, "men should investigate diseases in particular." But how?

In turning from speculation to actual observations, those who followed Sydenham's lead took a scientific step forward. But the only type of observation which Sydenham urged was that of the bedside— maladies were to be distinguished simply by their symptoms. Much effort was expended during the 1700's in attempting to do this. Some of the more obvious diseases were better described, and a few new entities—such as lead poisoning—were discovered. But symptoms and their various combinations were numerous and confusing. When every particular symptom-complex was called a distinct illness and these names were compiled and classified, the result was a list of some 1800 so-called diseases. At this point, confusion became worse confounded.

Obviously, the physician could find little help in a "nosology" text that listed 1800 names as diseases. What he needed was a simpler guide to common maladies. This very fact led most medical men to hold on to the traditional humoral concept, which indicated a few traditional remedies. Others were tempted to think out other theories, each of which oversimplified matters by postulating some underlying condition basic to all illness.

Clues to such theories were found in each new discovery and this made the most speculative hypotheses appear up-to-date and "scientific." Thus, when chemists distinguished between acids and alkalies, it was promptly suggested that sickness of every sort must result from either too acid or too alkaline a condition in body fluids. And, in this case, all the practitioner needed were a few acid or alkaline remedies.

Illustrations of this trend are afforded by the speculative use of circulation and of Haller's research on the physiology of nerves. These centered attention on the branching networks of the vascular and nervous systems, and it was quite naturally assumed that anything which went wrong with these would react upon the entire body. Could not the state of blood vessels or tensions in nerves account for almost any symptoms? Such reasoning, however "modern" it seemed at the time, simply revived the ancient *strictum et laxum* pathology of the solid parts.

About 1760 William Cullen, a medical professor at Edinburgh, began to emphasize the role of nerves and blood vessels in producing illness. Then a Scottish student of his, one John Brown, declared that all disease resulted either from tension or laxity in the vascular system. This meant that one could forget the innumerable species of diseases listed in nosological texts and just treat these two general conditions. If the patient's troubles were due to hypertension, he needed to relax and Brown gave him laudanum for this purpose. If he suffered from the opposite condition of flabbiness, a "tonic" to build up the tone of muscles and nerves was indicated. And there was Scotch whiskey right at hand as the best tonic imaginable. So Brown's followers dosed their patients alternately with laudanum and with "Scotch" and one can understand why these treatments were popular in some social circles.

Another pupil of Cullen's, Benjamin Rush of Philadelphia, brought this viewpoint back to America and there carried it to its logical extreme. He eliminated lack of tone as a cause of sickness, and so reduced every illness to the one condition of hypertension in the blood vessels. He was convinced that he had thereby solved all the problems of pathology. More than that, he had settled all questions in therapeutics; for now all one needed in any case was a single procedure that would reduce tension. This he found, not in laudanum, but in bleeding. Could not anyone see that if you bled a patient long enough, he would always relax—sooner or later? And so the Philadelphian advocated, for patients who did not relax easily, the removal of as much as four-fifths of all the blood in the body!

Rush was very proud of what he called his "system" of pathology and treatments, and made it by 1800 the most popular one in America. Meanwhile, other system makers agreed with him that there must be some basic, pathologic state, but disagreed as to what this might be. The majority still held that it was the condition of the humors, but others thought it was the state of some one organ such as the stomach or the brain.

If one system-maker was right, all others must be wrong; and, as a result, each engaged in controversies with his rivals. They carried these debates into lectures and even into the newspapers. Since they were all equally dogmatic, educated laymen—seeking "enlightenment" —came to wonder whether any of them really knew what they were talking about.

The quarrels of medical men thus hurt the reputation of their own profession, which now compared unfavorably with that of physical scientists. A few critical physicians joined with similar laymen, by 1800, in declaring that medical science was lagging behind amidst general progress, and that some fresh start must be made.

Continuing Developments in Medical Research

The expression of such protests was in itself a good sign, and recalls that there was another side to the medicine of the 1700's than that which has been emphasized so far. For one thing, some real research continued in pathology amidst all the speculation noted.

It will be recalled that anatomists already pointed a way out of the confusion of nosology texts. They had suggested that lesions found at autopsy could be correlated with ante-mortem symptoms, so as to identify a limited number of diseases. In this way, one could recognize specific illnesses and abandon generalized theories, and at the same time not have to think of innumerable symptoms as all constituting diseases in themselves. Studies of this sort involved careful bedside observations as well as autopsies, and could be pursued only if the proper facilities were provided.

Such facilities never became adequate during the eighteenth century, but they were somewhat improved by two social developments. First, the public authorities in some Continental countries—Italy, Holland, Austria—were by this time willing to permit autopsies on poor patients who had died in hospital wards. It was chiefly in the English speaking lands, by 1800, that the public still opposed autopsies or even dissections for teaching purposes. British and American physicians could rarely secure "subjects" for dissection except by robbing the graveyards. And this led to "doctor's riots," when mobs tried to attack medical men and to wreck their laboratories.

In the second place, the growth of commercial or manufacturing cities necessitated the building of larger hospitals. Here were increased opportunities for both clinical observations and autopsies. These were not extensively used before 1800; but a few medical leaders began to follow their fatal cases to death houses in order to see what light could be thrown on the diseases involved. They realized that hospitals, planned originally for charitable relief, had unintentionally provided them with research opportunities not available in private practice.

If a religious order provided nursing in a given hospital, the Sisters continued to view their patients as "God's poor," but research-minded physicians came to look upon the same people as so many cases for investigation. This was a "hard boiled" attitude; but, in the long run, it held possibilities for science and therefore for human welfare.

The first fruits of these enlarged opportunities were, once again, to be observed in Italy. At Padua, where a tradition of anatomic research had been maintained since Renaissance days, Giovanni Morgagni checked the symptoms observed in wards with the lesions found at autopsies. The number of patients observed at any one time was still small, but Morgagni kept careful records for almost fifty years. Finally, in 1761, he published his great work on "The Sites and Causes of Diseases." The title was significant. Diseases were localized in particular parts and could be identified thereby. He gave, for example, the clearest accounts of aneurysms and other vascular lesions yet available, and showed that one should suspect such conditions in living patients. Here was a program for an anatomic instead of a speculative pathology.

Despite the impressiveness of Morgagni's work, it was not widely imitated at the time. Practitioners remained indifferent as heretofore, since the description of disease processes provided them with no new remedies. Dr. Brown and Dr. Rush later proclaimed their speculative theories just as if Morgagni had never written. Even those medical professors who were anatomists failed, before 1800, to follow the Italian's lead much further than he had carried it. As in his case, their hospital "services" were only beginning to grow in size; and they probably lacked his patience in accumulating data over many years.

Morgagni's work and viewpoint gradually became better known, however, and were in due time taken up and pursued more intensively. This would come about when, by 1800, larger numbers of ward cases became available and when—for reasons to be noted later—physicians made up their minds to exploit these more effectively. The way for all this, and therefore for an end to the long dominance of speculative pathology, was prepared during the last years of the eighteenth century.

Developments in Surgery and Obstetrics. Preventive Medicine and the Beginnings of Health Insurance

Also on the credit side of the eighteenth-century record were certain advances in the practical branches of medicine. Such fields as surgery, obstetrics, and hygiene dealt with tangible matters, and so were less apt to be confused by theory than were pathology and therapy. One did not have to speculate about a fracture, a delivery, or the need for fresh air and exercise.

Surgery, during the 1700's, witnessed no improvements as basic

as those earlier introduced by Paré. But there was a gradual refine-
ment of such old operations as those for cataract and for "the stone."
A better knowledge of anatomy made a few new operations possible,
as in providing the earliest surgery for aneurysms. Dental surgery
received for the first time the attention of able men in contrast to that
of itinerant tooth-pullers. Better extracting instruments were contrived,
although what should be done after teeth were removed was quite a
problem. The only false teeth yet available were not really "false"—
they were those of animals or of other men who were willing to part
with theirs for a price.

As surgery acquired a scientific basis in anatomy, the prestige
of surgeons rose. Their guilds were separated from those of the barbers, and they gradually were associated with physicians in hospital
practice—to the advantage of both groups. In America, the two professions were merged from the start, since in a new, sparsely settled
land each practitioner had to serve many functions.

No great advances were possible in surgery, nevertheless, as long
as the humoral or tension concepts persisted in pathology. If diseases
resulted from impurities in the humors, for example, what was there
for surgeons to do? Who could operate on the blood or bile? Only
when the localized pathology of Morgagni was generally accepted,
would surgeons be called upon to remove diseased parts. Until that
time, surgery necessarily remained an art on the periphery of practice
and was employed only in case of such emergencies as fractures or
the removal of superficial tumors.

No such difficulty presented itself in obstetrics and here real
progress was made during the 1700's. Better knowledge of the anatomy
of gestation and delivery enabled physicians to handle difficult cases
more intelligently than could the midwives. The latter were trained
simply by apprenticeship and their folk art was adequate for only
normal deliveries at best. Some of them were disreputable creatures,
as immortalized by Dickens in his portrayal of "Sairey Gamp" in
Martin Chuzzlewit. Certain physicians, as a result of their growing
knowledge, became interested in obstetrics and correspondingly critical of the Sairey Gamps. The maternity and infant mortality rates
were very high and many of the deaths were clearly the fault of
ignorant attendants. A few innovators therefore advocated the service
of regular physicians or surgeons in difficult deliveries.

Here they ran afoul of the prevailing notion that, as a matter of delicacy, only women should provide obstetrical services. It had always been a woman's art. Much ridicule and abuse were heaped upon the first English physicians who were so brazen as to become "man-mid-wives." The French court had introduced a vogue for employing surgeons as "accoucheurs" before 1700; but in England, where prudishness seemed to increase, popular scruples were harder to overcome. Here was another illustration of social obstacles to technical progress.

Nevertheless, Dr. William Smellie introduced French procedures into London after 1740; and eventually he trained nearly a thousand men, as well as many women, in an improved art. Dr. William Shippen of Philadelphia, returning from Edinburgh, gave the first lectures on obstetrics in America in 1762; and he led a movement here to transfer the art to regular practitioners. Gradually, when professional leaders advocated the change, the upper classes in England and America came to accept it. Only poorer folk continued, because of conservatism and poverty, to employ midwives.

This victory of learned medicine over folk practice is usually celebrated as a triumph of science over prudery. But there was a less fortunate aspect of the matter; namely, the tendency to deprive women of their one, remaining role in medical practice. The midwife of 1700, with all her faults, represented a primitive professional type which—like the early deaconess—was half practitioner, half nurse. She could have kept up with improved methods if she had been given better training; indeed, this did happen later in some parts of Europe. But in English-speaking lands, for reasons unknown, this was not the outcome.

There is no doubt, however, that there was marked improvement in obstetrics in the hands of some physicians. Remarkable was the work of certain British leaders, whose common-sense demand for cleanliness anticipated later aseptic procedures. Special lying-in wards or hospitals were set up in the larger British cities, and in these it was shown that both maternal and infant mortality could be sharply reduced by proper care. The London Lying-In, for example, maintained in the 1790's a maternal rate as low as the average figure in many present cities.

Closely associated with efforts to safeguard maternity was a movement to check the high death rate among infants and young children. Books relating to pediatrics had appeared as early as the 1500's, but they became more common after 1700 in both Europe and Latin America. In London, for example, Dr. William Cadogan published an *Essay Upon Nursing* in 1747, and this aroused enough interest to go through several editions. Cadogan urged that all who nursed small children should follow a common sense hygiene. Infants should no longer be wrapped in swaddling clothes. These were picturesque, as one can see in the superb della Robbia medallions, but they probably appealed more to artists than they did to the babies.

There were other strange procedures. "The general practice is," observed Cadogan, "as soon as a child is born to cram a dab of butter down its throat. . . . It is the custom of some to give a little roast pig to an infant, which, it seems, is to cure it of all its mother's longings." Prosperous families turned their infants over to wet-nurses, sometimes with unfortunate results. And, once weaned, the children were denied fresh fruits and vegetables for fear that these were dangerous.

Poor children faced additional hazards. Illegitimacy was common, and great numbers of children in both Great Britain and Continental countries died of neglect or were murdered and then reported as "overlaid." This does not mean, however, that conditions were necessarily becoming worse. The protests which were made at the time indicate rather a growing concern for child health. Such concern, expressed through better care and medical attention, helped to bring about a significant decline in child mortality between 1750 and 1800. Combined with a continued high birth rate, this inevitably made for an increase in the total population of Western Europe.

Here was a beginning of the most marked population growth in recorded history, and physicians therefore had a hand in one of the chief social phenomena of modern times. Whether or not the whole trend was desirable was a matter of opinion. The saving of young lives seemed, in itself, an obvious gain. But even before 1800, an English thinker—Malthus—warned against the danger that soon there might be too many mouths to feed.

The infant welfare movement related chiefly to better food, clothing, and general care; that is, it was a drive for sensible hygiene rather than a matter of medical science. As such, it was one phase of a larger trend toward better rules of living in general. Adults, as well as children, needed such protection.

Some of the hygienic "enlightenment" of the 1700's was unplanned, such as the enlarged food supply that came with commercial expansion. But as people became "better off" and better educated, they consciously sought for higher standards of living. Once it was possible to live in a fairly clean manner, for example, cleanliness became of more concern in principle. Hospitals had long been content with "bug hunters" who just kept vermin down to a reasonable minimum; now they desired to have their wards entirely rid of such infestation.

Meantime, the upper classes even began to take baths. They also worried about their daily habits—about the effects of gluttony, drunkenness, or lack of exercise on the health of the individual. They therefore looked to physicians for guidance in the "rules of life." Manuals on personal hygiene became popular, and more was published on the subject in the 1700's than had been during the entire two preceding centuries.

Valuable as personal hygiene could be, few expected that it would prevent the greater part of illness. Hence it seemed that something more than hygiene was needed. Were the masses able to get medical care? If not, this was not only inhumane; did it not also threaten the interests of business and the State? The new industry needed healthy workers, and the national Government could not be strong if most of the population was sickly. In a word, economic developments and the growth of national feeling provided additional motives, in this age, for concern about the people's health.

Various schemes were proposed for national health systems which would assure medical care for everyone. One clue as to what might be done was provided by the beginnings of health insurance. Since the masses were unable to pay for the services of practitioners when ill, could not they save up for this purpose by carrying insurance? The principle of such protection had long been applied to marine insurance, and was being improved at this time by the development of better actuarial calculations. And by 1750, the British Government was already requiring certain groups of workers to carry hospital insurance.

Consequently, in the late 1700's, a number of reformers urged that the Government require all workers to take out insurance against the costs of medical fees and of hospitalization. No such system was actually introduced in Britain or elsewhere at the time, but the idea of compulsory health insurance would be revived during the next century.

The same era which witnessed efforts to improve personal hygiene and to provide medical care for the masses, was also a time of increased concern about what was termed "public health." The supposedly contagious diseases seem to be declining after 1750; for example, leprosy had almost disappeared, plague had ceased to invade Europe, and smallpox (as will be noted) was coming under some control. Fear of contagion therefore lessened, at the same time that concern for general cleanliness was mounting. Was there not some connection between the filth of the slums and the "fevers" and other diseases which plagued these areas? If so, sanitary reform rather than quarantines was the best means for preventing epidemics. Streets should be cleaned, and water and sewage systems provided.

Little was actually accomplished along these lines before 1800, but the demand for such a program was mounting. In this, as in so many other ideas of the late eighteenth century, men were reviving classical ideals. Greeks and Romans had always ascribed epidemics to bad local conditions—to "airs and waters"—and had therefore trusted in sanitary controls.

The revival of the classical view on sanitation was, in turn, part of the larger search for "enlightenment." The upper classes were becoming informed on the latent possibilities of science and of a secular outlook. These developments were believed to promise safer, more comfortable and more intelligent ways of living than had prevailed during the Middle Ages or the Reformation. Hygiene seen against this background was more than a branch of medicine; it was an aspect of civilization in itself.

Developments in Drug and Diet Therapy

Last but not least among the medical advances of the 1700's was the introduction of certain of the drugs or other practices of folk medicine. These were empirical in origin; that is, they had been stumbled upon over the years and just found to be effective. No one knew who had discovered these things or how, just as no one knows when or how folk music or folk tales originated. Learned physicians had long scorned popular remedies but some of them became more open-minded during the enlightenment era. Hence, when common folk reported a wonderful cure, a doctor here and there would look into it. What was found was often disappointing, but now and then it proved of really great value.

As a matter of fact, the only two specific drugs known during the 1700's—mercury against syphilis and cinchona bark (quinine) against malaria—had come into use from folk lore during the preceding centuries. But nonspecific drugs which affected general body processes (stimulants, sedatives, purges and so on) were also useful, and some of these were taken up from folk practice during the period 1600–1800. Thus, when Dr. Witherington of London heard of an "old woman" who could cure "dropsies," he examined her concoction of herbs and decided that its valuable component was the plant foxglove. From this was isolated digitalis, which did relieve dropsy (fluid accumulations) by stimulating heart action and thereby improving the circulation.

In such ways, a few drugs of value seeped into the pharmacopoeias that had been published in various countries since about 1600. At first, these compilations contained only a little sense in a great mass of nonsense. There was no exact way, as yet, of determining whether or not a drug was valuable. If patients recovered after using one, the drug was given the credit and went into the pharmacopoeia. Hence the latter included many supposed remedies which had accumulated over the centuries.

Most drugs were plant products, which had little or no value but did no harm. Mineral and metallic drugs (mercury, antimony) were also coming into use after 1600 and these were sometimes dangerous. Likewise employed were various animal concoctions—lice, crab's eyes, worms, excreta—which seem to have been valued in proportion to their repulsiveness. By the later 1700's, however, most of these obnoxious preparations were eliminated.

In addition to remedies, folk lore also contributed ideas or processes calculated to prevent illness in the first place. Seamen, for example, had long known that scurvy did not occur as long as a diet of fresh meat and fruits was available. But such foods were hard to keep on long voyages or, for that matter, to have at hand on land during the winter season. Scurvy, in consequence, was a common and serious disease. Looking into the possibilities of a protective diet, medical officers of the British Navy confirmed the reputed value of fresh fruit; and thereafter the disease could be prevented by carrying supplies of citrous juices. All this was empirical knowledge, but it anticipated the rational understanding of vitamins that would come more than a century thereafter.

The use of a protective diet was more a matter of specialized hygiene than it was a medical measure. But the first strictly medical procedure intended to prevent disease was likewise brought into practice from folk lore. This was the custom, long followed by peoples in the Orient and in Africa, of inoculating healthy persons with the poison (virus) of smallpox. The person so treated contracted the disease but usually in a mild form, and was thereafter immune to the infection. Knowledge of the practice reached Europe, 1700–1720, from Turkey and from China; while Americans heard of it from their African slaves.

Inoculation was risky, since deaths occasionally followed; and it did seem a strange business to deliberately "give" a dangerous disease to a well person. When fatal smallpox epidemics visited London and Boston in 1721, however, fear became so great that experiments with inoculation were undertaken. This was done with only a few cases in the former city, but was tried with over 200 persons in Boston. Curiously enough, nearly all physicians opposed the practice, while the leading clergy supported it. The great issue was: Were the dangers of death greater if one was inoculated, or if he waited to take the disease "in the natural way?"

Assuming that nearly everyone would acquire the infection sooner or later (which was true under the circumstances), the answer was in favor of inoculation. The death rate following that operation was only 1 to 2 per cent, while the rate in natural cases ran as high as 15 per cent. This was shown by keeping figures on the results—one of the first instances in which medical conclusions were reached by statistical methods.

Inoculation thus prevented fatal results in this much dreaded disease. The process therefore represented the beginnings of preventive medicine—more specifically, of immunology—and this was a milestone in medical history. Inoculation slowly spread thereafter, despite much opposition, throughout Europe and America. Then, in 1799, the English physician Jenner showed that cowpox "virus" could be used instead of smallpox, with results that were much safer and equally effective. This modified form of inoculation was called vaccination and has been used ever since in order to prevent smallpox.

Like other folk practices, inoculation and vaccination were empirical measures; no one understood how they operated. As far as smallpox was concerned, it was enough just to know that it "worked." But the lack of theoretical understanding made it difficult to apply similar processes to other diseases. Why not inoculate people also with the "viruses" of measles, tuberculosis, or syphilis, in the hope of getting mild cases and subsequent immunity?

Actually, such experiments were made but with discouraging results. Not enough was known about these particular diseases, or about immunology in general, to warrant such action. (Imagine inoculating all the youth of France with syphilis, as was seriously proposed in Paris shortly after 1800.) Yet the basic possibility of preventive medicine was established in 1721, and meantime smallpox itself was brought under some control.

Professional Standards of Medical Practice

While medical science and practice exhibited, in the abstract, such gains as have been noted, what of the professional groups which actually carried on the medical program? During the 1700's, the functions now maintained by physicians were still divided in Europe between a number of guilds—between surgeons, apothecaries, midwives, and physicians proper. The latter constituted the elite among practitioners; they alone were really "doctors" because they had taken university degrees. (Only in the English American colonies, where there were no universities to give degrees, were all practitioners called "doctors" as a matter of courtesy.) Physicians belonged to the upper classes and were patronized by the gentry.

In earlier centuries, physicians could attain fame and fortune best by serving the nobility or high officials of State and Church. But as the middle classes also acquired wealth between 1600 and 1800, the opportunities for fashionable practice became greater. Fees were given for individual services, and those paid to prominent doctors became quite high during the 1700's. The all-time record in such matters was probably that established by a Dr. Thomas Dimsdale, who received about $50,000, a title, and a pension for inoculating the Russian royal family against smallpox.

When physicians were paid in cash fees they naturally desired to make money, and the same was true of surgeons and apothecaries. But the desire for income could not be reconciled easily with the older ideal of serving those in need. Indeed, physicians were pulled three ways: they must make money, they were supposed to give help when and where it was needed, and a few of them desired to contribute to science.

To some extent all three of these interests could be reconciled, as when a prominent physician gave free service to the poor in hospitals, used his patients there as subjects of study, and then secured an income through high fees to the rich. Some progress was made along each line—that in science and the acquisition of wealth have already been mentioned. A gesture toward further aid to the poor, meanwhile, was made by opening dispensaries where prosperous physicians provided drugs without charge. The example of English dispensaries was followed in America, after 1750, by those established in New York and in Philadelphia. These are of some interest, in that they may be viewed as the prototypes of later out-patient departments in hospitals.

Yet the interests noted were often in conflict, one with the other. The physician who strove for a fashionable practice usually did little for research and made only a gesture towards aiding the poor. And the true research man begrudged the time he had to give to making a living out of practice. Meantime, the quest for fees introduced an increasingly competitive spirit into medical practice. One physician was pitted against another, and all physicians against the rival guilds of midwives and apothecaries. It might be said that doctors acquired a split personality—part business men, part humanitarians.

In consequence general practice was in a most confused condition. Doctors indulged in the tricks of the trade to secure their rivals' patients. They also tried to ban from practice all who were not "regular" in the sense of meeting the licensing requirements of each country. In England, for example, the College of Physicians of London had the sole right to license physicians and granted this privilege only to graduates of English universities. Hence there was friction with graduates of Dutch or Scottish universities who tried to practice in England. But these groups combined could not provide for the mass of the people. The poor depended upon folk remedies, quacks, or self-trained "empirics," and some of them were admitted free in the hospitals of large towns. There, as charity patients, they also could see real physicians. Middle-class patients, not wanting charity and unable to pay high fees, secured medical advice and drugs from apothecaries.

In a day when dosing was the most common treatment, it seemed easy to ask the apothecary what to take. (Americans will still request druggists to prescribe, using some such phrase as: "What's good for a cold, doc?") And as apothecaries came to handle ordinary treatments, their guilds included in their training program some medical instruction. Finally, in a parliamentary act of 1815, apothecaries were authorized to conduct general practice but to charge only for their medicines. This encouraged much prescribing and gave the English a reputation as "those hard-dosing Islanders." Eventually, apothecaries gave more attention to practice and less to their shops, and then another group known as "chemists" began to sell drugs. These became "druggists" in the American sense.

Competition between physicians and apothecaries was common in France and in other Continental countries, as well as in England. This did not help the reputation of either guild and medical men were viewed quite generally as a quarrelsome lot. It is only fair to add that trouble between practitioners involved more than mutual rivalries. Just because practice was so uncertain in its results, one man could honestly believe that another was killing his patients; and controversy was almost inevitable under these circumstances. On the other hand, little competition occurred between physicians and surgeons. The work of these two groups did not seriously overlap and they were, as noted, drawing closer together by 1800.

The professional situation was, as noted above, much simpler in colonial America. Practitioners or "doctors" in this country combined the functions of all the guilds: they gave medical advice, sold drugs, and practiced surgery. They also pulled teeth and, after about 1790, took over midwifery for good measure. Few states required a license to practice and none demanded any formal training. In short, almost anyone who wished could practice medicine in America.

If the standards of practice were to be raised, both in Europe and America, much depended of course on the way in which future practitioners were trained. In the Old World, each guild had its own tradition in this regard. Those seeking to become physicians went to university medical schools, apothecaries and surgeons provided their own guild schools, while servant-nurses and midwives learned only by experience. Most significant was the training program for physicians, and this calls for further comment.

The advent of scientific studies in hospitals, already noted, was associated with basic changes in medical education. Here one must recall that physicians who were prominent enough to be professors in medical faculties were also appointed to the staffs of hospitals. As professors, they had long lectured on theoretical principles, while as staff members they just tried to relieve patients by traditional methods. But until the Renaissance, they had seen no direct connection between these two roles; students wanted theoretical learning and rarely visited the hospitals where only practical procedures could be seen. Medicine was learned from books (as law is today); that is, until about 1600, "library medicine" was in vogue. Practical observation could come after the student took his degree.

When medical professors began to *study* cases in hospitals, and not just to try to cure them, the situation gradually changed. Lecturing about particular diseases, for example, professors realized that it might help the students to see these diseases diagnosed in living cases. Therefore, they began to "demonstrate" such cases to students in the wards—the beginning of clinical teaching.

Italian medical schools had given students bedside instruction as early as the 1500's. The idea spread to Dutch centers during the next century, and was adopted generally in the better European schools by the 1700's. "Library medicine" was no longer enough; it should be supplemented by "bedside medicine."

This does not mean that clinical teaching was done on a large scale, since the hospital "services" available for this purpose were usually limited to a few beds. Nor was much time given to such instruction, for professors still found it easier to lecture than to demonstrate cases. The fact remains that hospitals began, for the first time, to be centers of education as well as of research; and these functions could be expanded whenever desired.

The results of this trend were somewhat different in England than in other parts of Europe. Oxford and Cambridge universities were located in small towns without hospitals. Hence, when clinical teaching was desired, students had to go to London to find it. Informal medical schools grew up in the hospitals of that city, where students "walked the wards" in order to acquire experience. In Scotland, however, the outcome was different. The medical school at Edinburgh, for example, used local hospitals and remained a part of the University. Hence British "colonials" in America had a choice when they first set up medical schools; they could copy either the English or the Scottish institutions.

During the 1700's, most Americans who sought medical degrees abroad went to Edinburgh. So they followed that model when they founded their first medical schools in Philadelphia and in New York before the Revolution. These pioneer schools were each connected with arts colleges which at least claimed to be universities (Pennsylvania and Columbia). Subsequently, however, many English-type, hospital medical colleges were also founded in this country; and a few of the latter, such as Jefferson in Philadelphia, still survive.

While medical education was slowly improving, professional life was enriched by the appearance of societies and journals. A few medical bodies, like the London College of Physicians, had originated in the larger cities during Renaissance days. These were select, guild-like groups, which had no contact with the rank and file of practitioners. During the latter part of the eighteenth century, physicians began to form medical organizations of a more inclusive nature. (The first in the United States was the New Jersey medical society of 1760.) Their purpose was, in part, to replace the long defunct guilds. They felt the need of bringing doctors together so as to lessen the bitterness of competition and to provide some rules for the game.

Dr. Thomas Percival, of Manchester, finally published in 1803 a famous code of ethics which was followed by most British and American societies. He stated the rules of professional courtesy and at the same time reviewed the broader obligations of physicians to the public. The one theme related to the doctor's income and prestige, the other to his traditional idealism. The professional quarrels of Percival's day led him to emphasize points of etiquette, while genuinely ethical questions were not stressed. There were, for example, admonitions against stealing another man's practice. This resulted eventually in some ridicule of professional ethics as "trade union rules"; but whatever phrase is applied, the code was of real service. Even the public benefited, in the long run, by efforts to inhibit jealousies within the profession.

The morale of physicians was heightened when they came to-gether in medical societies. There, also, they could exchange ideas about science and practice. Such communication went further when it was possible to discuss things with the world at large through publications.

Books, of course, had been printed since the Renaissance, but it was expensive in both time and money to get out an entire volume. A partial answer to this problem was the journal. The success of early newspapers after about 1680 showed that periodicals were possible, and several professional journals appeared in France and in Italy before 1700. But not until after 1750 did such publications—including some devoted entirely to medicine—become well established. The first American medical periodicals were the *Cases and Observations* of the New Haven Medical Society (1784), and the *New York Medical Repository* (1797–1824).

The importance of these developments can be realized if one tries to imagine physicians getting along today—as they had to do in 1700—without any professional societies or journals. By the time that lay nursing attained a recognized status after 1870, the need for such institutions would be commonly recognized; hence organizations and publications were made available in this field without long delay. In this, as in other respects, modern nursing was indebted to the earlier experience of the medical profession.

Summary

In summing up the story of eighteenth-century medicine, one must admit that no such progress occurred in this field as was evident in the physical sciences. The problems faced in the former were com-plex and obscure, those in the latter relatively simple. Hence, in medicine, the key science of pathology continued to be theoretical and confused; the true nature of disease remained an enigma. Even the advances made in sciences basic to pathology—anatomy and physiology —were seized upon for further and useless speculations about the

215

supposed nature of disease. The only encouraging development in this area was the continued search for a localized, anatomic pathology which might identify specific diseases, and this effort unfortunately made little impression before 1800.

On the other hand, there were real gains of a practical nature amidst all the theoretical confusion. Surgery and obstetrics were improved, and folk lore contributed new remedies and the beginnings of preventive medicine (inoculation). As aspects of general enlightenment, moreover, both personal and public hygiene received increasing attention; and a conscious child-welfare movement was associated with the first marked decline of the general death rate in recorded history.

Meantime, medical men began to improve their own institutions —to provide modern educational methods, societies, and journals—and so prepared themselves for a greater role in the future. These gains, technical and professional alike, were no mean accomplishments. Yet they were to be overshadowed by what lay ahead in the nineteenth century.

Chapter XI

The "Dark Age" of Hospitals
and Nursing

The history of hospitals and of nursing during the eighteenth century was influenced by the trends just described. The development of medical research and the growth of humanitarianism each played its part. As leading physicians began to pursue hospital studies, they became more active in these institutions. In Protestant England, where the Church had passed largely from the picture, lay boards gradually restricted their activity to finances and general policy. Physicians meanwhile acquired more influence in the wards and directed the nurses in medical matters.

Similar trends could be observed in the large municipal hospitals of Catholic countries, as in those of Paris and Vienna. The Sisters therein remained under ecclesiastical discipline, but in the treatment of patients were directed by doctors much as in Protestant countries. This transfer of medical matters to physicians was of distinct advantage as far as teaching and research were concerned.

On the other hand, there were disadvantages in professional control from the viewpoint of nurses and patients. In England, for example, women were practically eliminated from positions of authority in hospitals. The matron, although exercising some oversight over servant-nurses, was herself untrained and poorly paid. In consequence she tended to become subordinate to governing boards and to the medical staff.

It was also in English hospitals that other decadent tendencies, associated with the suppression of nursing orders, became most manifest. Poor wages, unpleasant drudgery, and the loss of religious prestige produced a deterioration in hospital personnel which became extreme by about 1750. The inferiority of personnel inevitably expressed itself in poor nursing and administration. How the sick poor were left to the care of old charwomen, some of them habitually drunken and dishonest, is an oft-told tale in all accounts of nursing history. To make this specific, the experiences of one of the English semi-public hospitals may be briefly recalled.

The London Infirmary was established in 1740, by a little group of benevolent business and professional men. Between them, they raised several hundred dollars and appealed for further aid to noblemen and other "subscribers." A meeting of all those who contributed regularly became the governing body (board), operating through an executive committee. This is worth noting, since it illustrates the type of management which became so common in Great Britain and in the United States.

Here was neither a religious nor a municipal establishment, but rather a private organization serving the public on its own initiative. The governments of English-speaking countries were especially inclined to "let well enough alone" in society as a whole; that is, to practice a so-called laissez faire policy. As a result, private activity was responsible for the origin of hospitals, schools, museums and other institutions of a sort which were supported by governments in Continental Europe. The Anglo-Saxon procedure had advantages in that it provided freedom of initiative, but the lack of government aid or regulation was sometimes a handicap in other ways.

But to return to the London Infirmary. Having raised a small sum, the founders rented a house and appointed a physician, a surgeon, and a "chemist" (druggist). The three were to visit the Infirmary each morning. Then a man and his wife were hired to look after the place and the patients. Between them, these two were to fulfill the duties of superintendent, steward, nurses and servants. After a year or so, it was decided that a nurse was necessary; so they employed a person called "Squire" who was not even honored by the title of "Miss" or "Mrs." She lived out and was paid five shillings a week. Several similar women were later employed, including "night watchers." This necessitated a head nurse or matron and the hall-door porter's wife was elevated to that station.

The records show, as might have been expected, a series of difficulties with this pathetic staff. Squire, the account reads, was reported to have taken money from patients; she was not dismissed, however, as "it was not in the rules that she should *not* do so." Another nurse, it was found, refused to give any service without tips. The matron practically starved the patients, so as to use funds provided for food for her own purposes. Several nurses were dismissed for drunkenness. Disturbed by this time, the executive committee (governors) raised the nurse's wages a little and advertised "for a sober, *grave* person, who is capable of acting as a nurse." Apparently none appeared. Had anyone applied, they would have certainly been depressed by the accommodations. A committee of subscribers, appointed as "house visitors," found that "the nurses receive their friends in the room in which the watches sleep, to the disturbance of their rest"; and it was ordered that thereafter "nurses should receive their acquaintances in the kitchen."

The patients also presented problems. They were kindly referred to as "the miserable objects"—which no doubt they were! Occasionally they were drunken and troublesome. More often their friends caused confusion by crowding in, bringing forbidden food and interfering with the servant-nurses. The smuggling in of food is understandable, when it is recalled that the miserable objects received only "water gruel" or "milk pottage" for breakfast, either boiled meat or boiled pudding for dinner, and for supper more "milk pottage." No other food was "allowed on any account whatever." It is interesting that neither physician nor surgeon saw anything objectionable in providing this one monotonous diet under all circumstances.

Perhaps the constant need for economy had something to do with this indifference. No doubt this also explained the provision of only one pair of sheets per bed, which leaves the matter of their washing something of a mystery. Sanitary arrangements were necessarily primitive. When the frequent filling and emptying of the cesspool became expensive, it was decided to let this "drain into the other cesspool *under the arbour.*" From here the contents overflowed into a neighbor's garden; and when he complained, that was settled by just renting the garden. Five years after the founding, when some seventy patients were being cared for, *one* cold bath was provided. Certainly there was no disposition to pamper the "objects," save in one respect. Convalescents were permitted to go out during the day and frequently just disappeared. One can understand that, too.

The London Hospital was not a minor, neglected place, but a permanent venture that became one of the great hospitals of the city. Conditions were actually worse among the sick who were stranded in public institutions other than hospitals. Jails were appalling places in both Europe and America, what with the lack of decent food and clothing, the filth, overcrowding, and general promiscuity. Prisoners who became ill, including the perfectly decent debtors, lay on dirty straw and were tended only by such of their fellows as were so inclined. The workhouses or almshouses established in English-speaking countries after the Reformation, were by the 1700's in almost as wretched a condition as the prisons. The larger ones had infirmaries attached, but nursing therein was performed chiefly by old paupers who were detailed for the purpose. The history of American almshouses like "Blockley" in Philadelphia and Bellevue in New York shows how drunkenness and insubordination were to be expected under these circumstances.

On the face of things, the chief objections to nurses were of a negative character. They simply neglected their charges and created a demoralizing atmosphere. But it should be noted that such men and women—for men were used in male wards—might also do positive harm. Some had the instincts of quacks and would try out remedies of their own, or withhold prescriptions of which they did not approve. They had their own notions derived from folk practice which progressive doctors found it hard to supplant. There was a popular conviction, for example, that fresh air and clean linen were dangerous for smallpox patients until the pustules had dried. Like so much folk medicine, this was a survival of earlier professional opinion which physicians themselves had abandoned after Sydenham's day. Many doctors found their efforts to secure clean clothes for the victims systematically sabotaged by ignorant attendants.

The attitude of some professional men who attended hospitals did not help matters. Certain physicians and surgeons seemed hardened or cold-blooded in their relation to the inmates. From the present point of view, the eighteenth century was still a coarse and brutal age, despite the stirrings of conscience displayed by early reformers. In addition, the increasing tendency to view patients as cases rather than as individuals must have been disheartening. Complaints were also made about neglect on the part of clergymen, who were supposed to visit the wards and conduct services. To many a "miserable object," these medical and clerical gentlemen must have appeared as smug and indifferent as they did to the condemned prisoner in Oscar Wilde's *Ballad of Reading Gaol:*

> The doctor said that death was but a scientific fact,
> And every day the chaplain called, and left a little tract.

Toward the end of the century, when the spirit of social reform stirred in England, protests were voiced there against hospital conditions. One William Nolan published at London *An Essay on Humanity* (1789), in which he condemned the indifference of physicians, the coarseness of nurses, and the callous flippancy of medical students in the wards. The famous English reformer, John Howard, visited many jails and hospitals throughout Europe, and his descriptions threw further light on deplorable practices.

The very rules which some hospitals adopted to remedy matters revealed their previous shortcomings. After Howard had protested against the administration of the Royal Naval Hospital at Haslar, in 1789, the nurses there were ordered to leave no foul linen in the wards, to change sheets once every two weeks, to stop concealing the escape of patients, and to admit no friends to their rooms. Any who indulged in fighting or drunkenness were to be discharged.

There were meanwhile signs of deterioration in the hospitals of other European countries, especially in large, municipal establishments. The faithfulness of nursing orders, particularly where they were overworked and isolated, could not entirely prevent this. Perhaps certain of these groups had lost, by this time, some of the freshness or zeal associated with their foundation in preceding centuries. At any rate, John Howard, who provided the best picture of all European hospitals shortly before 1800, frequently reported on bad conditions in the wards. The old Hôtel-Dieu in Paris, despite the presence of Augustinian Sisters, was denounced as absolutely the worst he had ever visited in any land. It was dirty, noisy, and so crowded that patients were still huddled two and three to a bed.

Howard found the men's wards in Spanish hospitals, where no

Sisters were admitted, particularly objectionable. The inmates took snuff and spat continuously on the unwashed floors. There and in most Latin countries, he observed a "universal prejudice . . . against the free admission of air and the washing of rooms." Surgeons were not very squeamish in such matters, but at Brussels one told him that the air in the wards was "offensive beyond description." Howard was struck by the pallor of the Sisters there and elsewhere, and ascribed it to the closeness of the rooms and their secluded life. He concluded, in line with the new interest in hygiene, that: "air and cleanliness, and an abstemious diet, are of more necessary importance in hospitals than any administration of physic."

It seems unlikely that such overcrowding, dirt, and bad air had characterized the better medieval hospitals. These conditions can hardly have encouraged the better sort of people to seek employment as attendants, even under the supervision of Sisters. There is testimony from Italian hospital authorities that, by the eighteenth century, an inferior personnel had intruded into nursing service. This situation, which suggests the same trend which was observed in England, was viewed in Italy as a late and unfortunate development.

English Hospitals and Nursing

There was, to be sure, another side to this story. There were many hospitals on the Continent, and some in Great Britain, in which nursing and other conditions were relatively good. Little has been said of these in most modern accounts in English, perhaps because of an unconscious desire to sharpen the contrast with nineteenth-century reforms.

Indeed, there are so many *favorable* comments in Howard's writings that, if one concentrated on these, it would be possible to present a rather encouraging picture. He was impressed by the high, church-like halls in Italian institutions, which by preserving medieval forms did something to provide adequate air. Over and over again he praised the kindly and faithful services of the nursing orders. In Munich he found the wards neat and clean, and both the friars and Sisters of Charity dexterous and attentive. The ancient Hôtel-Dieu at Lyons was a model in every respect—clean, quiet, well staffed. A large hospital at Warsaw, housing eight hundred patients, was in excellent order. Great attention was paid here to the sick by the Sisters "according to their usual practice." And at Stockholm—in a Lutheran environment—the chief hospital was likewise clean, neat, and well administered. Even in Spain, Howard declared the women's wards were in good condition and the smaller hospitals maintained by convents were admirable.

The very fact that so many protests against bad conditions were made in the late 1700's, in itself suggests that improvements were under way. Men frequently protest because their own standards have risen, rather than because conditions are necessarily worse. Evils hitherto unnoticed or ignored are then condemned as unbearable; and later readers of these accounts are apt to think that things must have been going downhill. So it may have been with the hospital reformers of the eighteenth century. It seems likely that many European hospitals were in as good condition in the late 1700's as they had been during the preceding century.

The whole protest against poor nursing and administration in this era was, as already suggested, a phase of the Enlightenment. Conditions were undoubtedly bad in many cases and in certain instances became worse. An optimistic opinion then developed that things could be permanently improved. It was the same with enlightened opinion concerning slums, slavery, prisons, and other social conditions or institutions. Each reform began with a recital of "horrible examples"—often true, but not always without some exaggeration—and then went on to definite goals. So it was with the reform of nursing and hospitals, and these specific efforts should now be considered.

To begin with England, as perhaps the worst example, it may be noted that hospitals there reflected bad social conditions in general. The industrial revolution, coming first in Great Britain, produced slums which were among the worst in the world. This meant a depressed working population which imposed peculiar burdens on the semi-public hospitals. Eventually, the most striking reforms in nursing, like those in public health as a whole, were to come in England. This was not because that country had been progressive in the treatment of its poor; but rather because it was backward until things became so bad that sweeping changes simply had to be made. Much the same comment must be made on American developments.

Yet even in Great Britain and the United States the beginnings of a hospital reform movement can be observed as early as about 1760.

223

During the ensuing century, this movement went forward in all Western countries and exhibited the following features: (1) the establishment of new types of specialized hospitals; (2) the provision of more adequate buildings and equipment; and (3) attempts to improve nursing education and personnel. Each of these may be considered in turn.

Establishment of Specialized Hospitals

During the Middle Ages, different types of hospitals had been distinguished largely in terms of the groups they served. There had been establishments for the aged, for the clergy, for Jews, and so on. Medical science did not differentiate sufficiently between diseases—except in the case of leprosy—to warrant separate places for particular forms of illness. But as physicians began to distinguish clinical pictures more carefully, this gave the first impetus to specialized practice. No one wished as yet to be known as a specialist, for only quacks had hitherto given all attention to particular parts or diseases. But physicians gave special heed to certain types of illness and this encouraged the founding of specialized hospitals. This could be observed in London, where before 1800 there were foundling (pediatric) institutions, lying-in hospitals, cancer hospitals, and so on. In other cases, special wards were set aside for contagious diseases or other disorders.

One of the most interesting developments in this direction related to the care of the insane. The witchcraft delusion had largely died down after 1750, for the naturalistic outlook of the Enlightenment discouraged it. Men returned to the view that mental abnormalities constituted a type of disease and should be treated accordingly. But no clear mode of treatment was available. Physicians recalled what Hippocrates had said about the humors in relation to insanity, but ideas about the black bile did not seem helpful in dealing with the weird behavior of "lunatics." Then, too, a sort of repulsion against such people lingered over from the days of demonology and witchcraft. Mild cases wandered at large, the victims of local ridicule. Active cases were shut up at home or thrown into jails and almshouses. There, when violent, they were beaten or "ducked," and frequently held in chains. At Bedlam, in London, crowds went to see them as they did the animals at the zoo. Such pioneer studies of psychiatry as that of Weyer were rarely read by physicians, most of whom avoided the whole perplexing and unpleasant business.

The reforming conscience of the eighteenth century, however, responded to the mistreatment of the insane, as it did to that of other unfortunates. Individuals who looked into local jails were shocked at what they found. Meanwhile, a few physicians tried to describe the psychology of insane behavior. Towards the end of the 1700's these two forces, humanitarianism and science, converged in a demand for better treatment and a more careful study of the insane. Both interests indicated the need of special mental institutions, where patients could be placed under medical observation.

In England the pioneer reformer was a layman, William Tuke, who established the famous York Retreat. Here mental patients were given kindly or "moral" treatment with encouraging results. Tuke's interest was primarily humanitarian. In France, on the other hand, outstanding innovations were the work of a physician, the courageous Philippe Pinel. Having read both ancient and recent authors on mental disease, he secured opportunity for practical study when appointed physician to two of the old Paris hospitals. Each had wards or sections which housed insane patients. Pinel immediately urged that they be freed from chains and otherwise kindly treated, and in the midst of the French Revolution succeeded in bringing about this reform.

There was much fear at first that releasing "maniacs" would lead to trouble. The result was often the reverse. What it meant at the time to some of the victims can be illustrated by quoting the account of a single case:[38]

> People awaited impatiently the result of the experiment. One of the patients who was led outdoors and saw the sun exclaimed, "Oh, how beautiful!" He was an English officer who had been incarcerated for a period of forty years; no one had dared to come close to him after the day when, in an attack of fury, he had killed a guard. After two years of remaining calm, following his liberation from the chains, the officer was allowed to leave the hospital.

Pinel was not motivated simply by humane considerations. How could he study the patients' behaviour if much of their madness was simply due to confinement? They must be liberated for purposes of

[38] Quoted in Gregory Zilboorg and George W. Henry, *A History of Medical Psychology*, p. 323.

observation. Like other French clinicians of 1800, Pinel wanted to examine his patients carefully. He realized that the hospital provided the materials essential for psychiatric studies, just as it did for other clinical investigations. His method of keeping case records was in advance of the casual notes taken by most doctors and was eventually accepted as an essential procedure. He finally published a work on insanity, in which he admitted that little was yet known about different mental diseases—he classified them simply as mania, dementia, melancholia, and idiocy—and urged good care and further research. The beatings and neglect, the bleeding and the indiscriminate use of drugs, must be stopped.

Other physicians, here and there, came to share this view. In the United States, for example, Benjamin Rush published the pioneer American work on psychiatry. This was conservative in tone, but condemned the more brutal treatments and stressed a medical approach. That in itself encouraged provision for the insane in general hospitals or in separate institutions. The Pennsylvania Hospital set aside special rooms for this purpose after 1755, and the first American "insane asylum" was established by the State of Virginia about 1770. Not until after 1840, however, would such institutions become common throughout Europe and America.

Provision of More Adequate Hospital Buildings and Equipment

The second step in hospital reform was the provision of bigger and better buildings. There was marked activity along this line in both British and American cities during the 1700's. In London alone, six new general hospitals were constructed between 1720 and 1760, and several special institutions were added thereafter. Old establishments like Bart's moved into new quarters. In the United States, the first general hospitals in the modern sense—the Pennsylvania, the New York, and the Massachusetts General—appeared in that order between 1750 and 1820. All of these possessed excellent buildings for the period, which naturally followed British models. These dignified Georgian structures, with their improved facilities for light and ventilation, can still be seen in St. Bartholomew's in London or in the Pennsylvania Hospital at Philadelphia. There were parallel improvements in buildings on the Continent. In Paris, for example, the antiquated Hôtel-Dieu was completely rearranged during the Napoleonic regime. Objectionable wards were closed, and some buildings were torn down and replaced by more modern structures.

It was in this period that "hospital planning" became a serious joint concern of doctors and architects. The relation of general to special wards, and the quarters provided for staff and for service facilities, had to be studied in terms of the latest medical opinion. At the Hôtel-Dieu in Paris, the new arrangements provided special wards for contagious diseases, for maternity cases, and for the insane. The growing interest of medical staffs in dissections and autopsies expressed itself in the provision of rooms for these purposes. It could hardly be expected at this stage that "nurses' homes" would be provided—save where separate quarters were occupied by certain nursing orders—but in some cases improved facilities were set apart for nurses within the main buildings.

Not all of the new hospitals were as attractive as Bart's or the Pennsylvania. Some of them, by the later nineteenth century, would be condemned as cold, dark, and depressing. Yet when first constructed, they seemed modern and impressive. In any case, they were naturally cleaner than the old structures and attempts were made to keep them so.

One can hardly say just when or to what degree standards improved in such matters as diet, linen, and fresh air. These varied much from one country to another, or even from one hospital to another in the same locality. The necessity for economy in public or semi-public institutions retarded improvements along these lines. So, also, did the popular fear of fresh air. But it must be remembered that fresh air often meant cold air, since no buildings of the time had central heating.

Some attempts were made in the late 1700's to introduce special nursing equipment. Hitherto, the only appliances available for beds, vessels, and other utensils were those used in ordinary life. Glass and silver articles began to replace those made of tin. Oiled cloth for draw-sheets was introduced. Iron beds and hair mattresses came in. Tin cans filled with hot water were used as bed warmers. The old alcoves or curtains were abolished to insure better ventilation, although this meant a loss of privacy. The chief difference between such equipment and the modern was in the lack of materials made of rubber. These were not available until the vulcanizing process was invented in the nineteenth century.

Improvement of Nursing Service and Education

The improvement of nursing services, listed above as the third step in hospital reform, proved a very difficult matter. This was especially true in Protestant countries which had lost the nursing orders. Attempts were made to attract better attendants by slight increases in wages, as noted in the case of the London Hospital. This was well enough in itself, but the funds available were usually inadequate to make it a real solution. So long as nurses did the work of servants, moreover, many boards would have declined to pay more than servant's wages even if the money had been at hand.

The failure to find better servant-nurses could also be explained by the hard, unpleasant character of the work involved. A young woman, going into domestic service, ordinarily preferred the environment of a private home to that of a public hospital. The same thing was true of men. Not only did ward work mean confining drudgery, but it also required constant, intimate association with the dirtiest and most bedraggled humanity. Much is said of the kindness of certain doctors in treating these miserable objects; but, after all, the medical men did not have to live with them as did the nurses. One can still see the difficulty of getting good attendants, under such circumstances, in modern poor houses and prisons. Most of the scandals which occur from time to time in such places, reveal the indifference or brutality of their personnel.

It is a mistake, however, to assume that all nurses in the earlier period were disreputable. The Pennsylvania Hospital, for example, employed servant-nurses as did other Anglo-Saxon establishments, and sometimes bought immigrant girls (bond servants) for the purpose. But the governors were careful in selections and discharges, and seem to have secured better women from the start than the paupers who were used in the neighboring almshouse. Nor were the large English hospitals always unsuccessful in seeking women who, because of personal kindliness, were willing to give long and devoted service. Such persons were similar to a good "practical nurse" in the modern sense.

Many years later, when students were admitted to the first English nursing school in the 1860's, they were advised not to disdain the older nurses. True, some of the latter had been drunken and dishonest, but it was stressed that others had been devoted and unselfish in their labors. The medical staff recalled case after case, within their own memories, of women whom they had all admired. There was, for instance, Sister Rahere who between 1820 and 1860 gave forty years of faithful service and then bequeathed her entire savings—some £250—to the hospital.

In other Protestant countries, like the German Lutheran states, the loss of nursing orders created the same difficulties as those encountered in Britain and in the United States. Soon after the Reformation, efforts were made to meet this situation by reviving the early Christian role of the Deaconess. Some good woman, usually of middle age, would voluntarily devote herself to the sick in her community. The emphasis was on home nursing and suggests the modern public health nurse. In German and Dutch cities Deaconesses served in this manner, often as official representatives of the local Protestant churches. Not only the Lutheran and Reformed congregations, but smaller, more individualistic sects such as the Moravians and Mennonites—notable for their humanitarianism—were aided by such women. Although such Deaconesses did not serve in hospitals, their existence did help to keep alive the ideal of good nursing. This was fortunate, since the actual hospital nursing had fallen into the hands of servant-attendants similar to those in England.

In Catholic lands despite the fact that various nursing orders remained available, some concern developed about the character of lay nursing-attendants. These had been first introduced to take the place of convalescents or other volunteer helpers. The degree to which such persons actually cared for the sick seems to have increased during the later eighteenth and early nineteenth centuries. Then, as in Protestant countries, the long hours and other discouraging conditions made it difficult to find good people for the work.

Although it was claimed that neither the very young nor the old made as good nurses as did the middle-aged, certain hospitals like those in Milan began to train foundlings for ward duties. This arrangement had advantages in providing cheap and disciplined workers. But it also led to the exploitation of helpless orphans in terms of long hours and low pay—an exploitation which persisted in Italy into the nineteenth century. Probably the most overworked and abused

229

nurses were those in a few large municipal institutions, like the General Hospital in Vienna, where the restraining influence of religious orders was lost.

There seems to have been a growing feeling in Catholic as well as in Protestant Europe that women made better nurses—presumably because they were thought to be more conscientious and humane. As noted above, Howard found in southern Europe that the women's wards were in better shape than were those tended by men. During the 1790's, therefore, the Emperor of Austria—a "benevolent despot" who desired social reforms—substituted women for men as attendants in the male wards of municipal hospitals.

There ensued, for a time, considerable protest. Convalescent men in particular resented what they felt was the intrusion of a petticoat regime within their walls. Eventually, male attendants were retained for the heavier work and for the duties of the present orderlies, while women made the beds, did the washing, and so on. How much women actually improved the service is a question, since they were simply attendants themselves and were notoriously exploited by Vienna hospital authorities. Despite this, the precedent was established for using lay women in the wards of government hospitals in Catholic countries. Eventually, the orders of nursing Sisters also accepted this arrangement. In 1835 in Bavaria, for example, the Sisters of Charity (Vincentinerinnen) granted permission for the older, experienced sisters to tend male cases.

Beginning of Medical Interest in Better Nursing Care

While these limited attempts were made to improve nursing personnel by more careful selection, or by replacing men with women, a new element entered into the situation. This was the appearance, for the first time, of a *medical* interest in better nursing. Heretofore, the only concern voiced in this connection had been of a religious or humanitarian nature. But during the eighteenth century a few physicians, chiefly in France and in Germany, expressed the view that nursing was an important factor in the recovery as well as in the comfort of the patient. No doubt many an observing sister or clergyman had, through the centuries, realized this from long experience. But they were not in charge of the cases; while the doctors who were, had been naturally inclined to give all credit to their treatments.

It took some courage and insight for a physician to recognize that the nurse also made her contribution to the outcome. Although the first expressions of this view have sometimes been treated lightly, since they did not lead at the time to any striking improvement, the recognition of a medical role for the nurse was really most significant. All later attempts to improve her status were based upon such recognition and were, in that sense, secondary to it.

The origins of this view are probably to be found, in part, simply in sad experience. Evidence of the results of poor service may well have suggested what might be accomplished if only proper care were available. A more positive influence, however, was exerted by the contemporary enthusiasm for personal hygiene. The more one realized the importance of regimen in maintaining health, the more obvious was it that good care was also essential to recovering health. And the regimen of the hospital patient was in the hands of the nurse.

One of the first and clearest expressions of the nurse's role in healing—in providing medical as well as custodial care—appeared in the famous *Encyclopédie*. This many-volumed work, issued at intervals by French scientists during the later 1700's, expressed the ideas of the Enlightenment era and prepared men's minds for the French Revolution which was to follow. The author of the article on nursing discussed the many duties which this involved, noting all those long associated with the servant tradition.[39] But he sounded a relatively new note in stating, also, that the whole outcome of a case might depend on the quality of nursing. This occupation, he declared:

> is as important for humanity as its functions are low and repugnant. All persons are not adapted to it, and heads of hospitals ought to be difficult to please, *for the lives of patients may depend on choice of applicants.*[40]

Despite enlightened opinion of this sort in France, the major concern with nursing developed rather in Germany and in countries under German influence. Manuals on the subject had been issued there since the later 1500's, perhaps because of the Protestant need for instructing lay attendants. And during the eighteenth century,

[39] These duties included carrying food, tending fires, sweeping, bathing patients, changing linen, emptying vessels, accompanying physicians on rounds, handling dressings, suppressing noise, quelling disturbances, and burying the dead!

[40] See the article "Infirmier," *Encyclopédie*, etc., VIII (Neufchastel, 1765), 707. Italics not in original.

Germany became a center of the movement for hygienic reform. Since no industrial revolution had yet occurred and the business classes were correspondingly weak, the spirit of laissez faire was not dominant as in England and America. Consequently there was more inclination in Central Europe to view individual health in relation to public health, and the latter in relation to state control.

Johann Peter Frank and other writers on "medical police" outlined in detail just how all individuals should live, in order to contribute best to the total welfare of society. Even the hour when young people should retire was to be set by the government. These medical writers were fully aware of the dangers to health inherent in poverty, and felt that British and American authorities seriously neglected their people in this regard.

With such an emphasis upon state control of personal and public hygiene, the improvement of hospitals and nursing naturally received attention as a part of the whole program. General works on hospitals appeared during the last quarter of the century, such as that by Sannazaro published at Pavia (Austrian Italy) in 1793. The Italian professor noted that only recently had the medical significance of nursing been clearly recognized. This was most evident, he pointed out, in the current efforts to improve the instruction of lay attendants. Such a procedure was desirable, Sannazaro felt, in both Protestant and Catholic institutions; though he believed that the service of religious orders continued to be a mainstay of morale and faithful attendance. He was glad to observe, incidentally, that religious lines were no longer drawn as far as patients were concerned.

The activities which this author had in mind were those of a number of German hospital authorities who, between 1780 and 1800, began to give lectures to their nursing-attendants. The prime mover in this direction was Professor Franz May of Mannheim, who was convinced that poor nursing was a major cause of hospital mortality and that the service must be improved in the interest of the public health. He did not hesitate to use the term "murder" in describing current practices, particularly in relation to the care of small children. Convinced that publishing manuals was not enough, May decided—as he put it—to become a schoolmaster to nursing-attendants. In 1781 he presented to the Mannheim authorities a plan for a nursing school in connection with the hospital. The officials approved and advertised the venture in local newspapers, and a series of brief lectures was inaugurated for both male and female attendants.

Dr. May's talks were presumably similar to the instructions given in his own manual, which was first issued in 1782. In this he urged attendants to give conscientious attention to patients regardless of their means or religious affiliations. Nurses were reminded that their services were an important part of treatment and were warned against quackery. There was the usual discussion of routine in terms of diet, bleeding, and bathing; as well as an admonition to follow closely the directions of physicians and surgeons.

Most interesting was May's realization, unusual at the time, that nursing personnel could not be improved until the attendants themselves were better treated. He condemned the "slavery" in which they were held; and reminded everyone that it was to their own interest to have satisfied, well-trained and faithful nurses. It was even suggested that a servant be detailed to take care of the nurse's personal wants. If such treatment were provided, and only the better applicants accepted for his school, the German professor believed he could develop a service which would preserve lives throughout the Fatherland.

Although Dr. May had the support of civil authorities, his medical colleagues reproached him with encouraging attendants to indulge in medical activities. Such ignorant folk, it was said, were sure to bungle treatments. Whatever truth there was in this, the protest may also have revealed some fear on the part of physicians of nascent professional competition.

Fortunately, it was taken for granted that attendants in training must combine brief classes with experience in the hospital. Some of the first to attend lectures were already working in the wards. In this respect, the course of nursing education just reversed the history of medical education. Nurses had always been in sick rooms and now were brought, for the first time, into the class room. Medical students, conversely, had long been in the class rooms, and were in this period first taken into hospitals. Each group needed something of the experience hitherto reserved for the other.

Despite the alarm of Mannheim physicians, the medical activities in which May's students were expected to engage were very limited in scope. They handled dressings and bandages, gave enemas, and ad-

233

ministered prescribed medicines. Some of this was also done by doctors or medical students; and it is difficult to generalize as to how far such functions were delegated to nurses. Apparently this varied with time and place. Howard noted the presence of a woman attendant at an operation in Stockholm, and was impressed with the skill of the Sisters in Munich in carrying on routine bleedings. Some advances in surgery, and the decided improvement in obstetrics, called for a little more technical skill on the part of attendants.[41] This is significant, in that it anticipated the day when a revolution in surgery would profoundly affect hospitals and nursing.

May's program seems to have produced a somewhat improved nursing personnel and attracted the attention of progressive hospital authorities throughout Germany. Dr. Scherf of Leipzig expressed a hope that all Protestant cities, where nursing was in the hands of the ignorant, would follow this example. Pastors were urged to call Dr. May's book to the attention of their congregations. Similar instruction began to be given in other cities and further manuals appeared. All of these emphasized the need for better selection, by physicians, of those who wished to enter the service. And some sought to allay the growing opposition to male attendants—based presumably upon experience—by declaring that even a man, if properly instructed, could make a good nurse.

One of these works, that of Dr. J. G. Pfähler published at Riga in 1793, gave the most detailed directions with a simplicity that was well adapted to the needs of average attendants. Much of the care here described would be considered good today, and at the time it represented marked improvement over medieval procedures. Linens, for example, were to be changed without removing the patient from bed. The most distinct contrast with present routine related to bathing, which was restricted to the use of tubs. Those who were bedridden just had their faces washed, and no doubt stood the experience pretty well. The failure to proceed further with the ordeal is not to be ascribed to inability to work out a routine, but rather to limited facilities. As noted before, if we today had to live in rooms as chilly as those in northern Europe then were, we would understand the aversion to both fresh air and cold water.

41 Some of the eighteenth century nursing manuals, such as Robert Johnson's *Friendly Cautions,* etc.—one of the few English works (London, 1778)—gave more instruction on surgical and obstetrical procedures than on any other subject.

After instructing successive groups of attendants in Mannheim for fifteen years, Dr. May called his program to the attention of the learned world in a series of lectures at the University of Heidelberg in 1797. There, three years later, he was called to establish another nursing school. The students in this case were girls from twelve to fifteen years old; which seems very young until one recalls that in those days American boys went to college at about the same age.

Some of the schools which followed May's example experienced serious difficulties. One intended to train men in the Charité at Berlin failed to materialize for the simple reason that no students appeared. This illustrates the difficulty of getting desirable applicants —especially men—who could meet even the modest requirements. Other hospital centers seemed more successful, for example, that which Dr. May left behind him at Mannheim. There the physicians continued to give annually a short course of lectures. These were practical as well as theoretical in nature, and were connected with a month's special training in the hospital. The students were provided with board and lodging during the course. Upon satisfactorily completing it, they were given certificates recommending them to the public.

So it was that the first nursing schools were founded in Germany between 1782 and 1815. Their advent resulted from such converging forces as the aftereffects of the Reformation, the impact of scientific Enlightenment, and the German desire to regulate public hygiene. Nothing like these courses of instruction was to be found at the time in the France of Louis XVI, the Great Britain of George III, or the United States of President Washington. Nor can one imagine a university in any of the latter countries approving a course of lectures on the lowly theme of nursing, as did Heidelberg in 1797.

Unfortunately, the early German attempts to select attendants more carefully were not very successful. Fifty years after the first lectures were given at the General Hospital in Vienna, in 1812, the nurses (Warterinnen) there were still an overworked, ignorant, and depressed class. One reason that neither selection nor lectures could do much to improve this personnel was because the nursing schools had no effect upon the system of administering hospitals and supervising nurses therein. As long as domineering superintendents or physicians treated nurses as servants, superior women would not enter the service. It is also true that the actual instruction given by Dr. May and his colleagues was of the simplest nature; a few weeks of lectures on ethics and routine duties and a month's special training in the wards—this seems elementary at best.

Yet these observations by no means rob the pioneer nursing schools of all significance. In them it was first clearly established that lay persons should: (1) be selected as carefully as possible, (2) be given lecture courses integrated with hospital training, and (3) upon completing this work, be awarded certificates distinguishing them from attendants who had received no such preparation. These requirements were essential to further reforms in nursing which followed during the 1800's. Dr. May cannot be blamed for the fact that social attitudes prevented his program from coming to fruition in his own time.

Summary

One can summarize the whole story by saying that three basic steps had to be taken before lay nursing could attain its present general form. The first was the realization of the significance of nursing in medical terms. The second was the establishment of the first schools to train nurses to enact this medical role. The third was to improve such schools and to establish them far and wide as accepted institutions essential to hospital medicine. The first step was taken in several countries between 1750 and 1800, but most definitely in Central Europe; the second was made in Germany between 1780 and 1800; the third remained for the ensuing century.

The final advance could be made only after new social forces and further medical research could "take off" from the position which the Germans had reached in 1800. Professor May would have been surprised had he foreseen that biological studies would finally confirm an old theory of disease causation, which in turn would make nursing so technical that training would be obviously essential. He would have been more than surprised, had he known that lay women worthy of this opportunity would enter nursing only when the service was placed largely in their own hands. For the best-informed physicians of 1800 had heard little of bacteriology and even less of women's rights. Men with microscopes, and women who combined ideals with determination, would hold the future of nursing in their hands within another half-century.

Chapter XII

The Social and Scientific
Background of Modern Nursing:

1800 to 1900

The nineteenth century reaped what the eighteenth had sown. This was apparent, first of all, in basic economic developments. The factory system, having originated in England, spread after 1815 to France and to the United States and eventually to central Europe. Such expansion was made possible, on the technical side, by practical inventions of many kinds and by an increasing use of steam power. Not only were steam engines employed in iron and textile mills, but they also provided new transportation facilities which were needed in order to distribute factory products.

In the United States, for example, steamboats began running on the rivers after 1800, and locomotives upon roads of rails after 1835. This speeded up trade, made it possible to open new areas in the West, and so promoted the further growth of Eastern cities as commercial centers. Manufacturing and trade thus combined to promote urban growth. By 1850 cities of a size never dreamed of before, except in ancient Rome itself, appeared in every industrial country. New York, which in 1775 had had a population of only about 20,000, had increased to over 800,000 before the Civil War. Similar expansion occurred in Philadelphia, Boston, and Baltimore. Most spectacular of all was the growth of Chicago, which advanced from about 5,000 in 1840 to over 1,000,000 by 1890. On the other hand, where industry was not established—as in much of the Old South—there was no corresponding city growth. Charleston, South Carolina, which was almost as large as New York in 1775, increased to only about 60,000 in 1860.

Urban developments, although impressive in mere size, brought many social evils. The rapidity of growth made it impossible to provide proper housing or recreational facilities, and there were few attempts in the English-speaking countries to provide city planning. It also happened that, after 1850, architects abandoned the Greek tradition and revived medieval styles. The latter were too intricate and difficult for them at first, so that the buildings of 1850 to 1890 were often monuments to bad taste. The result of these trends was that manufacturing cities, particularly in Great Britain and in the United States, became ugly, sprawling monstrosities. The poorer people crowded into unsanitary slums which bred filth, disease, and crime, and even the upper classes were not entirely safe from the evil consequences.

The mortality rates of American cities mounted steadily between 1820 and 1860. So, apparently, did the incidence of drunkenness, crime, and general violence. Never were our cities more dangerous places than they were in this era. No wonder that country folk feared the big town as a place of evil. A popular song, referring to a farmer's visit to New York City, repeated the chorus:

> The Bowery, the Bowery!
> They say such things
> And they do such things
> On the Bowery!
> I'll never go there anymore.

Some suggestion of the seriousness of urban disease is provided by the death rate from tuberculosis, which reached over 400 per 100,000 in large American cities after 1850. In recent years, in contrast, this figure has been only about 15 per 100,000. In other words, the mortality rate for this disease a century ago was more than twenty-five times what it is today!

Tuberculosis was not the only plague of the cities. Other respiratory diseases, notably pneumonia, took a heavy toll. As there was then little control of infectious conditions, various "fevers" now rarely seen (typhoid, typhus, diphtheria) were more or less endemic and flared up at times in epidemic form. Most feared were epidemics of yellow fever and cholera, which devastated commercial centers at intervals. A yellow fever outbreak in Philadelphia, for example, caused a mortality of ten per cent of the whole population in one summer shortly before 1800. A similar mortality rate in that city today would result in over 200,000 deaths!

Malnutrition diseases were prevalent, notably scurvy and pellagra, and indicated lack of proper food among the poorer classes. (Fresh meat, fruits, and vegetables were often lacking except in summer.) The various malignant and degenerative diseases, now the chief causes of death, were also present. But their mortality rates were lower than today, chiefly because these are primarily the illnesses of later years and the proportion of elderly people in the population was smaller a century ago. Infectious diseases then took such a toll of children and young adults that relatively few people survived beyond the age of 50. Hence the number of individuals susceptible to the diseases of old age was quite limited.

Since many died before 50 and even before becoming adult, life expectancy at birth was low. Few statistics are available, but it is estimated that in 1800 the average person at birth could expect to live only about 32 years. This index of general health did improve slowly throughout the nineteenth century. It is estimated to have risen to about 41 in 1850 and to almost 50 by 1900. This improvement, which occurred despite high mortality rates in the cities, can be credited largely to rising living standards outside the urban slums. As agriculture, manufacturing, and trade expanded, food, housing, and hygiene all gradually became better—not only for middle-class urban folk but also for rural and small-town inhabitants. And for most of the 1800's, the great majority of Americans lived in rural areas.

There were compensations, moreover, even in urban growth. Wealth, accumulating in the hands of the few, was sometimes diverted into the support of churches, charities, and education. Hospitals necessarily expanded and provided potential opportunities for medical investigations. Indeed, science benefited in general, since great cities supported various scientific institutions which could not have been maintained in a simple, agricultural society.

It is also true that the middle and upper classes could escape some of the evils of city life. They lived in the better neighborhoods and eventually migrated to suburbs. This was, indeed, the great age of the urban middle classes—made up primarily of business and professional groups. They controlled economic life and their ideals permeated society. In business, they stood for free competition and against governmental "interference." In politics, they inherited the ideas of the American and French revolutions; that is, they favored manhood suffrage, civil rights (freedom of speech and press, religious freedom) and representative government. In theory, they also called for social equality—or at least, for equality of opportunity. These several ideals, although not identical, were fused in the general concept of "democracy."

The business classes had originally asserted democratic demands as a means for overthrowing monarchs, landed nobilities, and monopolistic guilds. After coming into power, however, the middle classes often interpreted democracy to their own advantage and failed to apply it to those less fortunate than themselves. There was continued discrimination against certain elements in terms of sex, income, and race. Thus, women were denied political rights and admission to business and the professions. "Equality," meantime, meant little to the poor in the slums, and was openly denied to slaves on the plantations. Yet the idea of democracy was in the air and could be appealed to by middle-class reformers or by the poor themselves. Hence, in demanding equality with those above them, the middle classes promoted an ideal which would be later turned against them by those still lower in the social scale.

Conscientious middle-class leaders, aware of the discrepancy between their ideals and actual conditions, strove earnestly throughout the nineteenth century to overcome "social evils." They inherited social reform movements begun in the 1700's and carried some of them through to partial or complete success. Thus, in the United States, the anti-slavery movement took on greater vigor after 1830. By 1861 it became a major factor in precipitating the Civil War, as a result of which slavery was abolished. This by no means ended discrimination against Negroes but it was an important step in that direction. An unfortunate by-product of emancipation, however, was the fact that many freedmen crowded into urban slums, and even rural Negroes lost such medical care as the masters had once given them. In consequence, Negro mortality rates since 1865 have been much higher than those among the whites.

Various other reform movements flourished in this country between 1830 and 1900. Their nature changed somewhat from what it had been in the preceding century. Early reformers like Thomas Jefferson had advocated social improvements in a rather calm and rational manner, but nineteenth century leaders became sentimental about the "causes" which they served. This change reflected a shift in the general outlook of the times, from the realistic attitudes of the Enlightenment era to the romantic temper of the 1800's. Instead of rational analyses, people relished appeals to their sentiments: they wanted to look upon life as a soulful adventure. Under these circumstances, social reform movements became suffused with emotion. Their leaders cited "horrible examples" of suffering rather than cold statistics. A good illustration of all this was the book *Uncle Tom's Cabin,* which did so much to stir up feeling against slavery.

Certain of the romantic reform movements had implications for health and medicine. Thus, the temperance drive began among doctors, who viewed drunkenness as a factor in disease. Taken over by clergymen and laymen after 1830, temperance became an emotional crusade and drinking began to be viewed as a sin in Protestant circles. This crusade probably did reduce the incidence of what is now—in a return to scientific attitudes—commonly called "alcoholism."

Some reformers became aroused by other threats to health besides drunkenness. Gluttony destroyed more men, they held, than did alcohol. Ergo, diet must be improved. Health would also be served by greater cleanliness, fresh air, and exercise. Some zealots believed that better hygiene could take the place of all medicine and they made their appeal a sort of secular religion. Thus one Sylvester Graham (still recalled in "Graham Crackers") preached that a better civilization would emerge if men would just observe his "rules of life" and stay away from the doctors!

Of special significance for nursing was the women's rights movement. Beginning in the 1790's, this also took on the character of a crusade. Although ridiculed by most men and many women, the early feminists organized conventions and demanded woman suffrage, equal property rights, and admission to the professions. Women's magazines appeared. Most influential of these was *Godey's Ladies Book* of Philadelphia which lasted until the 1890's, when its place was largely taken over by the present *Ladies' Home Journal.* The editor of *Godey's*, Sarah J. Hale, strongly supported the need for women in all medical fields. Replying to critics, she declared tartly in 1852, "Talk about this [medicine] being the appropriate sphere for man, and his alone! With tenfold more plausibility and reason, we say it is the appropriate sphere for woman, and hers alone."[42]

In 1850 Elizabeth Blackwell became the first woman to take an M.D. degree in this country. When the medical schools still refused to admit women, a number of "female medical colleges" were founded. Finally, in 1893, the Johns Hopkins School of Medicine became the first prominent institution to admit women as well as men.

The feminist movement meant more to women who aspired to become physicians than it did to those who wished to enter nursing. After all, nursing had long been a woman's vocation and it was not necessary to fight a way in here as it was in medicine. Nevertheless, the gradual improvement in the whole place of women in society indirectly benefited nurses as well as their sisters in other occupations. The old tradition of servant-nursing would give way more easily to a professional program, if women could establish their right to professional status in other fields as well.

Except for the anti-slavery crusade, all the movements mentioned were moderate in nature; that is, they did not aim at changing the basic social order. Temperance, women's rights, and health cults could be fitted into a capitalistic economy characterized by private wealth, business competition and the like. In short, these movements did not challenge middle-class control of society. Even the so-called labor movement, which promoted trade unions among workers, sought simply to secure better wages and working conditions within the prevailing economic system.

In contrast, however, a few radical thinkers—most of them middle-class in origin themselves—urged "the laboring classes" to demand a new type of society. They formulated a philosophy called socialism, according to which private wealth was to be abolished or minimized, the "means of production" (capital) were to be placed in the hands of the State, and governments were to operate all large-scale business

---

[42] Quoted in Thomas Woody, *History of Women's Education in the United States,* Science Press, Lancaster, Pa., 1929, II, 344.

in the interest of the workers. In 1848 Karl Marx, a German leader of this group, published a "manifesto" calling on his followers to seize control of each nation and to set up socialist governments. Ordinary reforms, he declared, would never bring the working people full equality—business men must be deprived of their power before this could be achieved. His manifesto concluded with the appeal: "Workers of the world, unite. You have a world to gain and nothing but your chains to lose!"

This revolutionary appeal was inspired in part by the bad living conditions among urban workers. Some Socialists claimed that the disease conditions in manufacturing cities proved that middle-class, capitalist governments would never provide the laboring classes with decent lives and opportunities. The latter must secure control of society for themselves and not depend on reform from above. This outlook secured support among some trade unions in Europe and strong Socialist parties were organized there before 1900.

Most of these parties sought to gain control of governments by peaceful, democratic means. Eventually, however, more extreme socialists ("communists") seized the Russian government by force at the end of World War I (1918), and almost wiped out private business and private professions. Since that time, even the practice of medicine and nursing in Russia has been directed by the State—all doctors and nurses receiving government salaries and serving under strict, governmental control. Even the time which a doctor can give to each patient is regulated there by official rules. In the Western World, in contrast, medicine and nursing—like the other professions—were destined to continue as free or voluntary callings.

The seizure of wealth and the control of business and professions by the Russian Government was the extreme result of a long trend toward increasing the powers of the State. In less radical form, the same trend had appeared in most countries in Europe and America during the nineteenth century. National-states—as distinct from city-states or principalities—had begun to form in Europe in the late medieval and early modern centuries; but it was not until the 1800's that these came to dominate all the Western World. The Germans, for example, were not united under one government (one nation-state) until about 1870. And only the Civil War decided that the United States were really "united" under one supreme government.

The motives for bringing small principalities or American "states" together in large unions were partly economic in nature. Business was aided if many different currencies, languages, tariff barriers, and the like were eliminated. (Even today, American travelers in Europe are irritated by the relatively large number of these obstacles which survive there.) Gradually, as people became used to larger countries with these advantages, they transferred their loyalties from the smaller to larger political units. Patriotism replaced provincialism—the Virginian became loyal to the United States, the Bavarian or Prussian, to Germany.

As nation-states emerged, however, they became involved in rivalries for trade, territory, power and prestige. After the French Revolution, most European nations followed Great Britain and the United States in adopting democratic governments—involving manhood suffrage, civil rights, and representative parliaments—but this did not lessen the tensions between them. Whole national populations, rather than just princes as heretofore, became friends or enemies as the case might be. And when rivalries led to war, ever larger armies were organized. With such forces and more destructive weapons, wars resulted in greater suffering both from disease in camps and from combat. This, in turn, called for improved military medicine and nursing.

During the Napoleonic Wars (1800–1815) military surgery became more skilful and field ambulances were introduced. But it was not until the Crimean War in 1854, when France and Great Britain blocked Russia's desire to seize Constantinople, that the sufferings of sick and wounded British soldiers inspired Florence Nightingale to improve military hospitals and to introduce women nurses therein. The next major conflict was the American Civil War (1861–65), and here again there was much unnecessary suffering as a result of unsanitary camps, poor military medicine, and inadequate hospital facilities. Before the war ended, however, better hospitals were built and female as well as male nurses were provided for them.

It may seem strange that modern, secular nursing began—in both Great Britain and the United States—in the military services. The need for good nursing was certainly more continuous and on a greater scale in ordinary, civilian hospitals. But the military need was more sudden and dramatic, and reformers could make a potent, patriotic

244

appeal on behalf of soldiers. Moreover, once a need for better hospitals and nursing was admitted, it could be ordered into effect more readily by military than by civilian authorities.

More than patriotism, of course, was involved in early attempts to bring trained women into nursing services. These efforts were also inspired by the increasing humanitarianism of the age. This spirit, already apparent during the preceding century, became more and more evident after 1800 and was the motivating force behind most social reforms. The sufferings of individual soldiers were no greater in these later wars than in earlier conflicts, but the public was now more sensitive to them and therefore wished to do something about it.

In 1859, it was made clear that humane feeling was sometimes as potent a factor as was patriotism. In that year, when Italy and France were at war with Austria, the international Red Cross was first organized as a body to care for the wounded on both sides of any conflict. The Red Cross, in the nature of the case, made no appeal to patriotism but rather one to common humanity. It was no accident that the era which witnessed this event, as well as the early efforts to provide trained nursing, was also that which saw the abolition of flogging, the improvement of jails, and crusades to prevent cruelty to children and to animals. Humanitarianism, like democracy and nationalism, was on the march.

A third factor which made clear the need for better nursing was progress in the medical sciences. As long as therapy was simple and largely routine—as in bleeding and purging—not much preparation was needed by anyone who served as a nurse. Even physicians, in the United States, often took no more training than could be secured through apprenticeship to older doctors. But when medical knowledge became more extensive and complex, a need arose for the better education of both physicians and nurses. Before describing the advent of trained nursing, therefore, it were well to recall the medical advances which made such nursing necessary.

Development of Modern Medicine

It is difficult to say when modern medicine first appeared, since much depends on what is meant by "modern." Many persons assume that it all began with Pasteur and the control of infectious diseases as late as 1875. At the other extreme, some would date the beginnings as early as the sixteenth century in connection with the anatomy of Vesalius; or in the seventeenth, when Harvey demonstrated the circulation and Leeuwenhoek discovered microorganisms.

Certainly, prior to 1800, modern scientific methods had been introduced (experimentation, measurement), and considerable new knowledge had been acquired. Gross anatomy was well known; something of the physiology of nerves, of respiration, and of the circulation was understood; and chemistry promised to throw further light on the nature of body processes. Several valuable drugs had been found (cinchona bark, digitalis, mercury), and a beginning had been made in preventive medicine in the form of vaccination against smallpox. There was much optimism about "modern progress," and some philosophers—to mention one, Benjamin Franklin in Philadelphia—looked forward to the conquest of all forms of illness.

This optimism was not entirely unfounded. Certain major diseases, such as leprosy and bubonic plague, had largely disappeared in Europe; and smallpox could be prevented after 1800. The crude death rate was falling in Western Europe, chiefly because of a decline in infant mortality. This decline resulted from improvements in hygiene and in living standards rather than from any specific medical measures, but it contributed to general optimism in an era of "enlightenment." Science seemed to promise all things.

Yet the physician of today would not have felt at home with the medicine of 1800. Doctors still had the vaguest notions of diagnosis, identifying most illnesses only by the most obvious symptoms or by the parts affected. Thus, they spoke of various "fevers," such as the continuous or the intermittent. There was also "brain fever," "scarlet fever," and "yellow fever"; to say nothing of "bilious fever." Moreover, all these conditions were ascribed to some one underlying cause, such as the state of the humors (blood, bile), or a tension in the circulatory system. This was the old, generalized pathology inherited from the Greeks. And to improve the state of the humors, or to relieve the tensions, physicians knew nothing better than to continue bleedings and purgings regardless of any particular illness which might be involved.

One can hardly decide whether this sort of practice did more good than harm. It had some merits. Physicians considered the more general aspects of the patient's situation—his strength, state of mind, family environment, and so on. With these things in view, the doctor could employ common-sense wisdom in prescribing rest, diet, stimulants, and personal encouragement. All this meant much to the patient which later, cold-blooded science could not provide. At the same time, bleeding and purging weakened many patients when they most needed strength. And, meanwhile, the doctor gave nothing of value against the particular illness involved. Except for cinchona bark and mercury, he had no specific remedies.

As long as such ideas and practice were in vogue, medical science could never make much progress. Physicians thought they knew the one "cause" of illness and one or two types of treatment deduced therefrom. What more was there for science to learn? No doubt it was interesting to discover additional facts in physiology but this science had not uncovered any means for preventing or curing disease. Hence it seemed to have little bearing on practice. As far as practical matters were concerned, most doctors thought they knew all the answers—for all time.

How, then, did medical practice ever escape from this vicious circle of ignorance and complacency? The means were finally supplied by research, it is true, but the mere accumulation of discoveries in anatomy and physiology would have not been enough in themselves. One could have learned much, for example, about the structure and functions of the lungs without finding a cause or cure of pulmonary tuberculosis.

What was needed, one can now see, was a new outlook on the central problem of medicine; that is, on the nature of disease. After all, normal anatomy and physiology are just branches of biology; they could be studied if there were no such thing as illness in the world. What is distinctive about medicine is its focus on illness—its concern with pathology. It was the old outlook in pathology (the belief in generalized states common to all illness) which had to be modified if medical science was to go forward. This was essentially a matter of ideas, but ideas in the long run may be more potent than particular facts.

Although most doctors of 1800 ascribed little importance to distinctions between one disease and another, the opposite view had long been held by some medical thinkers. The opinions expressed by the Englishman Sydenham about 1650, for example, have been mentioned; that is, that there are many "specific" diseases in the world and that these are as real and different from one another as are various plants and animals. And if each disease was distinct from the others, it probably had its own peculiar causes and means of prevention or cure.

If this view was sound, a vista of research opened before clinical medicine. How could the causes or cures peculiar to each disease be found, until the disease itself was recognizable? Ergo, the first task before clinical science was to identify the different diseases. This was no easy matter, however, and Sydenham's followers floundered for a century in trying to distinguish one disease from another simply by differences in the symptoms. Their search led, as noted in a previous chapter, to schemes for naming and classifying all symptom combinations; but doctors found long lists of this sort of little use in practice. Hence they preferred to go on thinking of all illnesses as varied expressions of one underlying humoral condition.

A way out of confusion was finally suggested by just those anatomic studies which most doctors thought of little value for internal medicine. Anatomists had originally sought to describe normal structures but they had inevitably found diseased (pathologic) structures as well. And there often seemed to be some relationship between the symptoms observed before death and the injuries (lesions) found at autopsies. Thus, structural damage was found in the lungs after a patient had suffered from a chest condition. Was it not likely that the lesions were essential components of the disease which had been present? If so, the disease could be identified by these postmortem findings as well as by the ante-mortem symptoms. Phthisis (consumption), for example, could be defined as the disease which produced tubercles in the lungs as well as a certain train of symptoms.

Suggestions to this effect had been made by a number of anatomists during the two centuries between 1600 and 1800. But it took a long time for their ideas to make much impression on the medical profession. Reports on morbid (pathologic) anatomy were sporadic and unorganized until the Italian Morgagni published a great work on the subject about 1760. Morgagni was convinced that disease processes were localized in particular organs and he correlated the damage done in them with the symptoms produced. Even then, however, most physicians were so accustomed to thinking of disease only as a general state that they failed to accept Morgagni's concepts.

Then about 1800, with apparent suddenness, physicians in Paris began to apply Morgagni's view in a systematic manner. They observed each patient's symptoms carefully and, in case of death, correlated these symptoms with the lesions found at autopsy. Leaders like Bichat, Laennec, and Louis insisted that diseases were distinct (specific) and located in particular organs or tissues. They announced that they would abandon all speculations about humors or tensions, and would simply examine the human body as objectively as chemists examined elements and compounds.

The "Paris School" was encouraged in this by the surgeons. The latter had always seen conditions which were plainly localized and structural (skin diseases, fractures, tumors), and one had only to project this outlook into the interior of the body in order to accept such a pathology for all diseases. If surgeons saw injuries on the surface, physicians would find them under the surface as well. Surgical views had long been ignored by the learned physicians; but surgeons were now becoming more skilful (what with greater anatomic knowledge) and commanded more respect. The Parisian physicians therefore associated with them on equal terms and were more open to their suggestions.

The French were also aided by improved working conditions. Unlike the ordinary practitioner, who saw only a few cases of any particular disease, the Parisian leaders were clinicians; that is, they served in hospital wards where enough patients were available to permit thorough investigations. Doctors had worked in hospitals for centuries but not in any systematic manner; they had treated individuals but had not seen these cases as so many research data. Fortunately, moreover, the Paris hospitals had become larger with the growth of the city and the general hospitals had come under state control. The French Government favored science, and reformed hospital administration so as to give the clinicians better opportunities. For the first time, hospitals became something more than charitable institutions: they evolved into centers of research.

To sum up, the apparently sudden appearance of the "Paris School" can be explained by trends long under way before 1800. Some of these were scientific, others social in nature. The decision to study human disease systematically was inspired by the success of such objective natural sciences as physics and chemistry. The concept of diseases as distinct entities, rather than as generalized states of the body, was derived from Sydenham and other earlier thinkers. And the idea that diseases could be identified by correlating symptoms with local, structural lesions, was taken over from both anatomists and surgeons. Last but not least, the hospital conditions essential to a research program were provided by social developments—by the growth of cities, the reform of institutions, and the favorable attitude of the French Government toward science as a whole.

Specific Developments in Modern Medicine

The results obtained by French research, between 1800 and 1850, were truly impressive. The whole spirit of medical science changed. Instead of debating theories about humors and tensions, medical leaders devoted themselves to patient, systematic observations in the wards and dissecting rooms. Questions were answered by the evidence rather than, as formerly, by arguments and oratory. And, as time passed, methods of investigation were improved. Autopsies were performed with greater skill and clinical observations made more exact. Thus, in order to record symptoms more carefully, Corvisart introduced percussion and Laennec invented the stethoscope.

So valuable was the stethoscope, especially in detecting chest symptoms, that it has remained ever since a sort of badge of the medical profession. This simple instrument—originally just a wooden tube—*could* have been invented centuries before. But as long as illness was conceived as a state of the humors, few doctors desired to examine particular parts such as the chest. Only when the concept of localized pathology was accepted was there need for physical examinations; and, when this need arose, instruments were soon developed to assist the process. Again, one notes, it was a new idea rather than any particular fact which opened up novel methods and procedures.

By the middle of the nineteenth century, other instruments were invented which aided the clinician's sight, much as the stethoscope aided his hearing. Notable were the ophthalmoscope and the laryngoscope. Eventually, 'scopes of one sort or another were devised for examining every accessible body cavity; and some of the more recent ones are connected with electric lights and even with surgical instruments. The greatest achievement along this line, of course, was the discovery of x-rays by the German physicist Roentgen in the 1890's. With these rays, it became possible to see into nearly all parts of the body.

Long before x-rays were discovered, however, clinicians were able to envisage to some extent what was going on in the living patient. Having usually found lesions following a certain type of illness, they could assume in later cases of the same type that similar lesions were present. And in this way, clearer pictures of disease—more exact identifications—gradually emerged.

Earlier physicians had spoken, for example, of a vague condition known as "inflammation of the chest." In some cases of this sort, clinician-pathologists now found at autopsy a consolidation of lung tissue. This was correlated with more carefully observed, acute symptoms, and the total condition was thereafter identified as pneumonia. In other cases, tubercles and cavities were observed in the lungs, following long and wasting illness, and this condition was identified as phthisis (consumption). In still other cases, no lesions were found in the lungs but there was inflammation of the surrounding pleural sac. This condition (also exhibiting distinct symptoms) was identified as pleurisy.

In like manner, vague "fevers" were broken down into fairly-well defined entities. Typhoid and typhus fever, for instance, were differentiated by the discovery that intestinal lesions were present in the former but not in the latter. The respiratory diseases and gastroenteritis received especial attention because they were the infections then most commonly seen in hospital wards. But pathologic anatomy also revealed less common diseases, as when lesions were discovered in the brain, the spinal cord, and the endocrine glands. Such findings later became the bases for the modern specialties of neurology and endocrinology.

In a number of instances, pathology suggested that conditions long thought to be different diseases were really only the one disease in divergent forms. Thus, Laennec found that the tissue lesions in lung tubercles were quite similar to those found in scrofula—a common disease of the neck glands. He therefore held that both consumption and scrofula were forms of the one disease, tuberculosis; and later research was to prove this correct.

French identifications of disease were so impressive that physicians from all parts of Europe and America flocked to Paris for training. Returning to their homelands, they set up similar hospital programs; and major research centers appeared after 1830 in London, Dublin, Vienna, and several German and Italian cities. To some extent, the British had developed pathology at the same time as had the French. It was in London, for example, that John Bright—in studying the kidneys—identified the serious disease ever since known by his name. Meantime, in Germany, medicine had been largely speculative in nature; but when French research was finally established there in the 1830's, it inspired a complete revolution in scientific outlook.

The Germans now undertook pathologic studies with great thoroughness. Earlier than the French, they applied improved microscopes to the examination of diseased tissues. Finding that tissues were always composed of minute, living cells, they concluded that disease processes were finally revealed in the character of these cells. Pathologic anatomy, which had begun with the examination of whole organs (Morgagni), had then moved on to that of component tissues (Bichat), thus finally concentrated on what seemed to be the smallest units of life. Staining and sectioning methods were evolved, so that the observer could distinguish the difference between normal and diseased cells. Led by the great pathologist Rudolf Virchow, this "cellular pathology" became dominant thereafter and continues to be essential today. It makes possible, for example, a differentiation between benign and malignant tumors.

Physiology was not as intensely studied, between 1800 and 1850, as was pathologic anatomy. One had to plan difficult experiments in dealing with body processes; little could be learned by merely observing them, as was done with anatomic specimens. Yet a tradition of animal experimentation had been inherited from the 1700's and was continued by a few investigators. The French physiologist Magendie, maintaining Descarte's view that the animal body was a machine, practiced vivisection in an extensive and rather ruthless manner. He analyzed certain involuntary functions, such as neural-muscular coordination in the vomiting mechanism. More outstanding,

252

however, was the work of his pupil, Claude Bernard, during the era after 1850.

During the next half-century, the concept of an animal machine (biophysics) was not as fruitful a one as was the parallel idea of the animal body as a sort of laboratory (biochemistry). Physics was making rapid progress at this time, especially in the fields of electricity and magnetism, and this would eventually have its implications for medicine. (X-rays have been mentioned.) But between 1850 and 1875, developments in chemistry seemed to have a more direct bearing on physiology. Early in the century, inorganic chemistry had been formulated much as we know it today in terms of elements and of equations for their various compounds. By 1850 a complex organic chemistry (that of carbon compounds) was also being developed. The analysis of compounds into elements was followed by the reverse process of synthesizing complex materials from the elemental ones. And the world was startled when a German chemist actually synthesized urea, thus proving that substances produced by life could also be made artificially. It began to look as if the body were indeed a complex laboratory.

Claude Bernard took over from here, applying chemical methods to the study of basic, physiologic processes. Particularly brilliant was his work on digestion; in the course of which he described the chemistry of the chief types of food (proteins, fats, carbohydrates) and the effects exerted on these by the several digestive fluids (gastric juice, pancreatic juice, saliva).

In the course of his studies, Bernard passed from the observation of normal functions to that of abnormal or pathologic processes, as when disease of the stomach or pancreas interfered with normal production of their digestive fluids. This research was a valuable supplement to that of the anatomists; for disease in living bodies usually involves functional difficulties. These may appear before tissue injuries are present, or vice versa. In either case, pathologic physiology becomes as essential to the understanding of disease as is pathologic anatomy.

Results of Medical Research

Impressive as were the results of medical research, from a purely scientific viewpoint, they were not of immediate benefit to patients.

Efforts to identify diseases held some ultimate promise of finding causes and cures—once the diseases were clearly recognized. But for more than fifty years, pathologists were so engrossed in studying particular tissues, cells, and functions that they almost lost sight of the body as a whole. Disease was thought to be so localized that little heed was given to old notions about the individual's "constitution" or general condition. Lost to sight, also, were the patient as a person and the possible bearing of his hopes and fears on his illness. The ward patient became, to clinicians, merely a "beautiful case" of this or that—only the disease he harbored was of prime interest.

Some treatments were of course given in hospitals and the sick presumably went there in the hope of being cured. But therapy was gradually minimized, as clinicians lost faith in old remedies. Bleeding, purging, and blistering had been supposed to relieve the body of impure or excess humors, and were given up when the humoral doctrine itself was abandoned. To prove that this was a sound decision, moreover, resort was had to another basic procedure of modern science; namely, to measurement (quantification). Louis, for example, compared the mortality figures for one hundred cases of pneumonia which were bled with those of a hundred which were not bled, and the statistics indicated that this ancient procedure was of questionable value.

Clinical statistics of this sort were also applied to the effects of using old drugs, with the result that most of these were found useless if not actually dangerous. In research centers, doctors therefore assumed a negative attitude toward therapy (clinical nihilism) and advised physicians not to "interfere" with the healing powers of Nature. The only remedy used in the Vienna General Hospital, about 1850, was said to be cherry brandy or something of that sort.

Such practice represented the other extreme from the heroic measures long used before that time. It had the merit of eliminating dangerous bleedings and obnoxious drugs, but there was little of a positive nature which could be offered in the place of the old treatments. It is true that chemistry began, after 1820, to discover drugs whose value could be proven. This was done at first by analytic work, as when French chemists isolated quinine as the active ingredient in cinchona bark. This substance proved a more effective remedy against malaria than was the crude bark. Various other active substances,

254

useful as laxatives, as soporifics, or as analgesics, were also isolated from vegetable materials during later decades. But no new "specifics" (drugs which would cure particular diseases) were discovered before 1900. For the most part, the best therapy involved simply a good regimen.

The fact that therapy was so helpless could not, in the long run, be concealed from the public. There was much criticism, in consequence, of the futility of medicine. Engineers were doing wonders with steam engines and telegraphs, but what were medical men accomplishing for mankind? In an effort to overcome such skepticism, certain physicians reverted to the idea of proclaiming one cause and one curative procedure for all diseases—much as the old theorists had once blamed all illness on the humors and credited all cures to bleeding. The German Hahnemann, for example, announced that each disease could be cured by drugs which produced the same symptoms as did that disease ("like cures like"). And an American, one Thomson, declared he could relieve all illness by vegetable compounds alone.

Encouraged by such promises, many sick persons abandoned "regular" physicians and patronized Hahnemann's followers (homeopaths) or those who called themselves "botanic" or "Thomsonian" practitioners. Late in the century, patients resorted to the "osteopaths" —a medical sect which ascribed most illness to spinal conditions and promised cures by manipulating the spine. These sectarians became groups which rivaled the regular physicians and did much to undermine public confidence in the orthodox medical profession.

The position of the "regulars" was difficult. If they went on bleeding and purging, the sectarians offered more pleasant remedies. If they abandoned bleeding and purging, could they admit that real science had as yet found few substitutes? Clinicians could be as nihilistic as they pleased; *they* had a captive audience in the wards. But family doctors had to satisfy critical patients. It was therefore most fortunate for them that medical science, at just this point, began to show practical results.

The first field in which the new pathology "paid off" was surgery. Progress therein has usually been ascribed to the discovery of anesthesia in 1844 but this is misleading. The value of inhalation anesthesia (with nitrous oxide) was actually discovered in 1799 but no one gave it any attention. The explanation seems to be that, as long as physicians ascribed illness to the humors, there was no need for surgery except for emergencies like setting fractures or performing amputations. After all, one could not operate on the blood or on other fluids. Acceptance of a structural pathology by 1840 changed the picture. If disease was localized in special parts, these might be repaired or removed and the source of disease eliminated. Surgery, it was now seen, could be most useful in internal medicine, and it began to move from the periphery to the center of medical practice.

Under these circumstances, more able men were attracted into surgery and efforts were made to improve its techniques. Hence, when the dentist Morton demonstrated ether anesthesia at Boston in 1844, the procedure was promptly adopted all over the Western World. Prior to that time, patients had been strapped down and remained conscious throughout the most painful operations; now they were rendered mercifully unconscious of the ordeal. The way was not yet open to major surgery because the risk of infection was too great; but emergency operations were rendered painless and the goal of more extensive surgical interference was in view. No one could deny that, in anesthesia, medicine had provided a real boon to mankind. This procedure, like vaccination before it, was just as practical as was anything produced by inventors or engineers.

Even greater usefulness for medicine, moreover, lay just ahead. Sydenham's faith, that the identification of specific diseases would enable science to find specific causes and means for prevention or cure, began to be confirmed during the last half of the nineteenth century. The first step, once a disease was clearly known, was to seek out its cause or etiology. And since the chief killers of this age were the infectious diseases, attention centered upon them. What enabled a disease of this sort to pass from one person to another; and, in cases of epidemics, to attack whole populations in dramatic manner? Some unusual causal factor must be present here, since epidemics were only occasional phenomena; and it might be easier to find such a factor than it was to explain chronic or degenerative diseases which were always present.

Epidemics had long been explained by two theories. One of these held that subtle poisons or "miasmata" seeped into the air from filth or decaying materials, and that these poisons spread disease wherever such air was breathed. This theory was dominant until as late as the 1870's, and it led to widespread fear of filth and insanitary conditions. A sanitary reform movement was aroused, and led to the establishment of permanent health departments which fought for clean streets, "pure" water supplies, and adequate sewage systems. Some good was accomplished; as when better water supplies encouraged cleanliness, and this in turn decreased the incidence of typhus fever which is born by body lice.

Sanitation, however, failed to check the spread of diseases which are now known to be conveyed by contagion. This was the second, traditional theory—that epidemics were carried by contacts between men or between men and animals. But what disease-principle, what inducing factor, might be passed from one man to another? Here, again, an old theory was recalled which might give the clue.

Ever since the 1600's, a few medical thinkers had insisted that infections were caused and spread by "little animals" (microorganisms). The behavior of epidemics could indeed be explained in this way but there was long no proof. Early microscopes were not powerful enough to observe microorganisms well. Moreover, as long as specific diseases were not clearly recognized, no one could search for the particular organisms which caused each one of them. The situation improved when better 'scopes were developed during the 1820's; thereafter, microscopic life was observed more clearly. Meantime, specific diseases began to be identified. Bassi, an Italian scientist, proved in the next decade that a plant disease was caused by a fungus. Why not human diseases as well?

By the 1850's, various medical men had observed minute plant forms (bacteria) in infectious materials taken from men or animals. Skeptics then declared that these organisms were merely the by-products rather than the causes of disease. But if bacteria were merely products of infection, they had not been present when the infection started; that is, these living forms must have been generated spontaneously from other materials. Was this possible? A negative answer was given by the French chemist, Louis Pasteur, who proved by laboratory tests that no bacteria appeared unless some were there in the first place. This made it seem probable that the microorganisms were not mere by-products of infection; they were more likely to be the original causes of this process.

Acting on this suggestion, Joseph Lister—a surgeon in Edinburgh —decided to destroy all bacteria which might gain access to surgical wounds. This he did about 1865 by spraying incisions with carbolic acid, which was known to kill microscopic life. The incidence of post-surgical infections, such as "hospital gangrene," immediately fell sharply. No one knew what organisms Lister was killing but the method worked.

It required another ten or fifteen years before the majority of surgeons in Great Britain and America adopted Lister's procedure; but once they did, surgery became far safer. The technique was later improved by sterilizing instruments and hands rather than by using carbolic sprays, and postoperative infections became even more rare. With both anesthesia and aseptic techniques available, surgeons could now invade major body cavities with relative safety. By 1890 abdominal operations were becoming common and the public was already talking of "the wonders of modern surgery."

Physicians dealing with specific, infectious diseases, however, faced a more difficult problem. They had to discover just what organisms caused a particular disease, if anything was to be done to prevent or cure that disease. Principles of proof were formulated and called "Koch's postulates," after the German bacteriologist who insisted on their application. The suspected organisms must be found in the sick person or animal, must be isolated and grown on some laboratory medium, must then be injected in a healthy animal and there produce the disease again.

It took time to develop techniques which would make these steps feasible; culture media had to be found on which bacteria would grow well, and dyes and staining methods had to be devised which would make one species of bacteria appear different from another. German bacteriologists solved these problems by about 1875; and in that year both Koch and Pasteur finally proved that the disease anthrax was caused by a species of bacteria called the anthrax bacillus. It seemed incredible that such minute organisms could injure and even kill large animals and men but there was no doubting the evidence. An old theory was finally vindicated after two centuries of skepticism.

The discoveries of Koch and Pasteur encouraged systematic efforts to identify pathogenic organisms and further discoveries followed fast. Between 1875 and 1900, bacterial causal factors were found for such common and dangerous diseases as typhoid, cholera, tuberculosis, pneumonia, and diphtheria. No "germs" were found for certain other infections, such as smallpox, yellow fever, and influenza; for the reason—we now know—that these are caused by viruses so minute that they could not be seen or filtered out at the time. But the search was so successful, on the whole, that it seemed as if all causal factors in infections would soon be uncovered.

Practical results also followed. As soon as cholera and typhoid bacilli were identified, for example, it was shown that they were carried chiefly in drinking water and at times in food. Public health agencies could therefore prevent these diseases by providing uncontaminated water, or at least by filtering or otherwise purifying the water before it was used. Other organisms, such as those of diphtheria, were found to be spread indeed by contagion, and this led to a revival of old notification and isolation procedures in the case of these particular infections.

Meanwhile, biologists discovered that some of the infections whose "germs" were not yet known—yellow fever, typhus fever, malaria—were spread by insects. If men could avoid these vectors they could escape the diseases even without knowing what organisms were involved. This information was especially valuable in the tropics, where yellow fever and malaria had long been major scourges. But all progressive countries benefited by a knowledge of insect vectors as well as of bacteria, and a new preventive program became possible. Health departments, instead of advocating hit-or-miss sanitation, began to know what particular steps had to be taken against each disease in turn. The "doctrine of specificity" was proving a spectacular success.

There were, nevertheless, some limiting circumstances. Diseases spread by contagion could be only partly checked by isolation; respiratory conditions, for example, continue to be conveyed in this manner at the present time. Further progress was made against certain infections, however, by the development of vaccination procedures. Pasteur observed that if an attenuated or killed vaccine (composed of specific organisms) was injected into an animal, no illness followed and the animal became immune to the disease involved. The vaccine was too weak to cause illness but aroused the body's resistance mech-

259

anisms, which remained alert against any future attacks by the same organisms.

The principle here was the same as that long employed in vaccination against smallpox, in which cowpox virus was used as an attenuated form of smallpox virus. But Pasteur knew the organisms with which he was dealing and could begin a search for other possible vaccines. Most dramatic was his preparation of one against rabies ("the Pasteur treatment"), as well as one against anthrax. Eventually, successful vaccines were prepared also against cholera, typhoid, yellow fever, and—in recent years—against poliomyelitis. In the case of diphtheria organisms, which produce a virulent poison or toxin, what amounted to a vaccine was made up of combinations of this toxin with neutralizing serum. Wherever the use of this "toxin-antitoxin" became common, diphtheria almost disappeared.

In due time, therefore, health departments were able to employ two lines of defense against infectious diseases. Sanitary controls could prevent any exposure whatever to infections like cholera and typhoid. Where exposure was unavoidable, men could be made actively immune by vaccination against such diseases as diphtheria and yellow fever. The combination of these preventive programs, as administered by health departments in progressive countries, helped to bring about a rapid decline in crude mortality and a corresponding increase in life expectancy at birth. In the United States, for example, such expectancy had been about 41 in 1850 and 50 in 1900. Thereafter, it rose rapidly to around 68 by 1955—an average life span which few would have believed possible a century before. Medicine was at last exerting a real influence upon society.

Since the greatest mortality decline was among children and young people (the age levels on which individuals were first attacked by infections) the percentage of those living into older years steadily increased. This brought complications, because more people lived to a time when they were exposed to the diseases typical of old age. Hospitals, after 1915, saw less and less of such diseases as typhoid and diphtheria, and more and more of the degenerative and malignant conditions. No certain means of preventing or curing most of these diseases were found, in part because in most cases their causes were not ascertained; and they remain the chief challenge to medical science at the present time.

Meantime, however, further progress was made against such infectious diseases as could not be prevented by either sanitation or active immunization. In such cases, could not cures be found? The first thought was that a specific drug might be discovered which would cure a particular disease. Quinine was known to be a "magic bullet" against malaria; perhaps others were waiting to be identified. This was an old idea, but most drugs which were known to kill bacteria would also kill the patient. Success against one major disease, however, was finally attained about 1910, when a German chemist—Paul Erlich—found an arsenical compound which would destroy the bacteria causing syphilis. This drug, salvarsan, usually did not injure the patient and yet apparently cured the disease.

The discovery of salvarsan led to a hopeful search for other specific remedies. No success ensued over nearly twenty years; but in the late 1930's, German chemists produced the sulfa drugs and French and British clinicians proved that these had curative effects on many hitherto resistant infections (pneumonia, meningitis, mastoid infections, and so on). Then, in the 1940's, another type of "wonder drug" was found in the antibiotics. These substances (penicillin, streptomycin, and many others) were usually derived from molds or soils, and were microorganisms which attacked pathogenic bacteria. They proved effective against a wider range of infections than did the sulfonamides; even tuberculosis responded to streptomycin.

Long before this, the clinical nihilism of 1850 had given way to a renewed confidence in therapy. The physician now not only had effective ameliorative drugs, such as analgesics, but he could also prescribe such curative procedures as surgery and the use of antibiotics. So promising were these remedies that there actually was danger of overdoing them. Some surgeons, between 1890 and 1920, were reckless slashers; and some practitioners in recent years have prescribed sulfonamides or antibiotics promiscuously—with serious reactions or "side effects" in some cases. But on the whole, therapy has been made vastly more effective during the last two decades.

Progress in preventive medicine and therapy was not entirely limited to the area of infectious diseases. Physiologists, studying the biochemistry of nutrition, discovered the role of the "vitamins" in preserving health. Serious malnutrition diseases—scurvy, beri beri, and pellagra—were checked by the use of these substances or by foods containing them.

In these cases, disease had been caused by the lack of substances needed from the outside environment in the form of food. But the physiologists found that illness was also caused by a deficiency of materials normally produced within the body itself. After Bernard had studied the glands which emptied juices into the digestive tract, other physiologists investigated glands which poured their secretions directly into the blood stream. Such secretions (hormones) were shown to have a potent effect on other organs and hence were dubbed "chemical messengers." Injury to any one of these glands, resulting in a lack or excess of its secretions, produced serious illness.

One instance of this was the fatal diabetes, which followed degeneration of certain cell groups (islets of Langerhans) in the pancreas. When the islets failed to secrete their hormone (insulin) blood sugars could not be utilized and metabolism broke down. A Canadian physician, Frederick Banting, finally was able to isolate insulin from the glands of animals; and it was found that diabetic patients could use such animal insulin in place of their own. The patients were not actually cured, but were without symptoms as long as the proper amount of insulin was supplied.

Somewhat analogous to the use of insulin was the discovery, a generation ago, that pernicious anemia could be controlled by the feeding of liver extracts. And in recent years, a hormone produced by the adrenal glands (cortisone) and one secreted by the pituitary (ACTH) have been found to suppress the symptoms of a number of diverse diseases—of rheumatoid arthritis, asthma, certain gastrointestinal conditions, and so on.

There was nothing specific about the action of the hormones. Certain of them seemed to be secreted in greater amounts in order to counteract any stresses to which the body was subjected, regardless of whether these stresses involved simply mental tensions (fear, anxiety), physical damage, or invasion by microorganisms. This fact has led pathologists to revive the older interest in the general state of both body and mind. Diseases, it is now known, are specific in some respects (typhoid vaccine will prevent only typhoid) but involve generalized conditions as well. The metabolism of the whole body is conditioned by a deficiency disease, and the complex called hypertension affects the entire circulatory system and eventually the organs most directly connected therewith.

Even the causation of disease was found to be a matter of general as well as of specific factors. True, typhoid fever never appears in patients except when they are invaded by typhoid bacilli. But some individuals who are exposed to these organisms never "come down" with typhoid. There is therefore some other factor present in susceptible persons, besides bacteria, which accounts for their "taking" the disease—something in the nature of weakened resistance. The blood is unable to develop effective anti-bodies against the invaders and this inability may result from poor general conditions. Thus, a healthy soldier remains immune to tubercle bacilli; but if subjected to undernourishment and exposure in a prison camp, his resistance is lowered and he acquires tuberculosis.

Realization of these circumstances has affected practice. Better food, reinforced by vitamins, may increase resistance to certain infections. In the case of tuberculosis, again, the best treatment until recently was simply to build up the patient's condition by rest and diet. In this as in other infections, the bacteria are not *the* cause; they are only one causal factor among others. General resistance may be so important, indeed, that in some instances—as in poliomyelitis— many persons are invaded by the organisms but only a few acquire the disease.

The revival of generalized pathologic concepts was encouraged, finally, by developments in psychiatry. Psychiatrists and neurologists sought, during the 1800's, to find brain lesions by which they could identify specific mental diseases. This was typical of the pathology of the time. In certain cases the search was rewarded; paresis was shown to be a form of syphilis, and senile dementia a form of arteriosclerosis. The first of these could be treated by salvarsan and, later, by antibiotics. Here were instances wherein the body clearly affected the mind. Recently, moreover, hope has appeared that drugs may prove effective against other types of mental disorders. But most mental illnesses showed no characteristic brain lesions, and psychiatrists turned about 1900 to a study of possible psychologic factors.

Most striking in this connection was the work of the Austrian psychiatrist, Sigmund Freud, who elaborated a theory that neuroses resulted largely from the social inhibition of sex impulses. These impulses, suppressed by the individual, were said to persist in his "unconscious mind"; whence they expressed themselves in the form of neurotic symptoms. Freud's method of treatment (psychoanalysis) was a purely psychologic, as distinct from a physical or somatic one. Widely adopted in some circles, it also influenced thought in literature and in the social sciences.

Psychoanalysis became a controversial subject, because it was difficult to prove or disprove its validity by the usual scientific methods. Whatever its merits, the original procedure requires so much time for each patient that it is difficult to see how it can be employed on a large scale. Psychiatry in general, nevertheless, has been influenced in one way or another by Freud's concepts and methods.

More important than psychoanalysis, for medicine as a whole, was increasing recognition of an old truth: that the mind influences the body in many ways in both health and sickness. If mental strain is prolonged, for example, a gastric ulcer may result; and if this is removed by surgery, some other illness will appear in its place. Remove the strain by psychologic or social guidance, on the other hand, and health may be restored. In such cases, the specific disease (the ulcer) is relatively unimportant; the basic condition is a generalized one known as a state of mind.

Mind-body relationships (psychosomatic medicine) are now of growing concern to clinicians. A consideration of them reveals, moreover, the limitations of the specific pathology of the last century. Intent only on the particular, localized disease, the clinician of 1850 or 1875 gave little thought to its mental implications. Although this approach led to great achievements, as previously noted, nothing was done for illness in so far as it involved mental factors. This may be a quite serious matter, as when anxieties or other tensions induce—or at least complicate—hypertension and heart conditions.

The old hospital practice not only ignored mental factors; it must often have made these even more acute. The whole treatment accorded ward patients—as helpless "specimens" in a strange environment—probably aroused fears which actually hindered recovery. In a word, generations of patients paid a price for those advances in specific medicine which now benefit posterity.

There is no need, today, for continuing to exact such a price. The good physician will consider not only the specific disease from which a patient suffers, but also the latter's general condition and his state of mind. So, too, will the good nurse. As just noted, the sick person's fears mount when he finds himself in a hospital, so that his mere presence there may complicate his illness. And at this point the nurse can do much to overcome his anxieties. Indifference or irritation on her part may threaten the patient's whole state; conversely, sympathy and encouragement—even in little things—may so improve an individual's morale as to aid his recovery. All this is true of the doctor as well, but the nurse sees more of her charge than does the doctor. Ask any former patient!

Meantime, even more than the patient's mental state requires the attention of medical men. This state, which may be a factor in the illness, has its origin in the sick man's personality and in his social environment. What influences have been exerted on him by his job, his family, or his general surroundings, and by his own particular reactions to these things? The investigation of these circumstances may call for cooperation from psychiatrists, social workers, or social scientists, just as the study of physical disease requires the aid of biochemists or pathologists.

In these and in other respects, physicians are returning today to the broad perspectives of earlier periods. But they return with knowledge rather than speculation about generalized conditions, whether these relate to physical, mental, or social phenomena. Such knowledge supplements that concerning specific diseases which was acquired during the nineteenth century. In consequence, present medicine possesses more penetrating understanding and more effective procedures than were ever available before in man's long history.

This does not mean that medicine has solved all its problems. Indeed, its very successes have created new difficulties. The mortality from malignant and degenerative disorders has increased over recent decades for the reason already noted; that is, more people now survive into the years which are subject to these diseases. To a large extent, such conditions are still unpreventable and incurable. In addition, many of those now saved by science live on only in a state of chronic ill health.

Despite the menace of these trends, the balance sheet of medicine shows gains on the credit side. No one would wish to return to a medicine so confused and helpless as was that of 1750, or to one so scientific and yet so ineffective as was that of 1850. Nor would most of us desire to see children and young people die from early infections, even though their survival means suffering from chronic illness in later years. Science, having met old problems, moreover, may at any time solve certain of those now confronting us. Certainly, it is better equipped for this task than was ever the case before. Achievement in the past gives some ground for optimism about the future.

Influences of Medical Advances on Nursing

Rapid advances in medicine and their useful applications led to social and professional repercussions. For one thing, public confidence in medical science and practice was restored. The licensing of physicians was made more strict and popular support of medical sects declined. Both governments and private philanthropy began, after 1900, to provide greater funds for medical institutions—for schools, for hospitals, and for research.

Meantime, scientific research inspired a general reform of medical education in the United States. New subjects and laboratory equipment were introduced in the medical schools, and their courses were extended to four years followed by a hospital internship. In this and other ways, the schools were more closely integrated with hospitals, where much of the training and research was carried on. As knowledge increased, specialties appeared in practice; and future specialists were trained in "residencies" after taking the M.D. and the internship. Hospitals thus became centers of graduate as well as of undergraduate medical education.

As word spread about more effective treatments, the public lost some of its fear of hospitals. Prior to 1890, it was largely the poor who were sent to these institutions for lack of home care; thereafter, those who could pay also sought admission—usually at the urging of their physicians. Certain subjective risks were involved for patients, as has been pointed out, and some might have been better off in their homes. But the hospital had two great advantages. It enabled leading physicians to see more patients than could have been attended otherwise. And it offered expert services, in terms of staff and equipment, which no single doctor could provide in the home. The more technical medicine became, the more true this was. No wonder that the expansion of hospitals since 1900 has been phenomenal.

What were the implications of this situation for nursing? And what influence did nursing, in turn, exert upon these developments? Prior to about 1860, those who tended patients served much as specialized domestics. They took care of rooms, beds, and the physical needs of patients, and had few medical functions other than giving routine doses of medicine. Even the better ones were rarely the equivalent of good "practical nurses" today. When clinicians introduced physical examinations, however, demands began to be made for a more skilful type of nursing service.

Beside the stethoscope and other 'scopes used chiefly by physicians, additional instruments were employed to aid in observing symptoms more exactly. By the 1860's, watches were being used to time the pulse and thermometers to measure temperature. Eventually, other measuring devices were introduced, such as the one for recording blood pressure which was invented late in the century. Nurses were asked to make observations with these instruments during intervals between the doctors' visits and to keep a record of the data. They were also expected to measure doses more carefully (hypodermic needles were invented about 1850); and to employ certain procedures (such as giving enemas) which required judgment on their part. Hence there arose a need for nurses who displayed more skill and reliability than could be expected of servant attendants.

The second circumstance which called for more intelligent nursing was progress in surgery. Operations, prior to 1880, were performed in homes as well as in hospitals, sometimes on kitchen tables and with only members of the family as assistants. The introduction of anesthesia, of aseptic procedures, and of complex instruments and techniques, however, gradually transferred most surgery to the hospitals. As the need grew for more careful handling of dressings and instruments, nurses were called upon to serve as operating room attendants. Greater skill was also expected of them in providing postoperative care. Training, as well as character and intelligence, was required for such services.

It was no accident that, just as these needs were arising between 1860 and 1880, the first training schools for nurses were established in Great Britain and in the United States. And when the early graduates of these schools entered hospital service, the clinicians found that they had the very qualities which were now needed in wards and in operating rooms. They were "just what the doctor ordered." If, on the other hand, surgery and internal medicine had still been as limited in 1880 as they had been in 1800, there would have been less need for trained nurses; and the graduates of schools would have had little advantage over practical attendants. The new type of nursing appeared in response to a new type of medicine; the two were well joined.

Subsequently, as medicine grew increasingly technical, the union between medicine and nursing became even closer. A broader training of nurses was indicated in order that they be kept up to date on the latest science. Some entered specialties which paralleled those in medical practice—qualifying for work in such areas as surgery, obstetrics, psychiatry, and public health. In the latter field, nurses often supplied general medical attention in neighborhoods or communities where the availability of physicians was at a minimum. Still others did "private duty" in homes or in hospitals, where patients or their families realized that good care might make all the difference.

It was in hospitals, however, that trained nurses were of greatest service. They became integral parts of the whole "medical team," and both the supervision and training of nurses became vital administrative functions of the larger institutions. Without trained nursing, indeed, hospitals simply could not have evolved into great centers of medical practice, teaching, and clinical research. Many of the technical advantages of recent medicine would have been lost, if their application had been left in the hands of ignorant and otherwise low-grade attendants. Hence, in recalling next the beginnings of trained nursing, one presents an essential aspect of the development of modern medicine as a whole.

Chapter XIII

The Emergence of Modern Nursing
in the Nineteenth Century

During the early decades of the nineteenth century, religious orders continued to provide nursing in the hospitals of Catholic lands. This service exhibited both the merits and the limitations which have already been described. Some adjustments were made to changing attitudes, as in the introduction of certain Sisters into male wards; and early in the century, some new nursing orders were established.

Notable was the appearance, in Ireland, of the Sisters of Mercy and of the Irish Sisters of Charity. The former, founded by Catherine McAuley of Dublin, began in 1827 as a secular group but adopted in 1830 the rule of the Presentation Order. They served in various Dublin institutions over the next two decades and then built their own hospital there. Meantime, they opened a house at Bermondsey in England; and in 1842 one of the group, Mother Warde, brought the Order to the United States. Here they established the Mercy Hospitals in Pittsburgh and in Chicago.

The Irish Sisters of Charity originated with Mary Aikenhead. After training in an English convent, she began nursing in Dublin homes in 1815; and later gathered other Sisters around her who did volunteer nursing in Dublin and in Cork (Cobh). In 1833, some of these Sisters received practical training in a Paris hospital and they subsequently secured their own hospital (St. Vincent's) in Dublin.

Gradually, they extended their services into other Irish institutions and even into their own foundation in distant Australia.

Toward the middle of the century, a number of nursing orders were established in the Church of England. This Church, it will be recalled, had not assumed responsibility for hospitals after the Reformation. But regret had been expressed, from time to time, that nursing Sisters were not available to the English people; and by the 1840's a "high church" (Catholic) movement within the Church of England revived an interest in religious orders. Several such Anglican groups were founded between 1845 and 1855, and these Sisters did general welfare work among the poor which included volunteer nursing during epidemics.

The first English order devoted entirely to nursing, St. John's House, was founded in 1848. This group established a training program in London hospitals, under which candidates served as "Probationers" for two years and then became "Nurses" who received board, lodging and small salaries. From the latter were selected, finally, a senior group called "Sisters" who could live either in the Order's Home or with their families. In 1861 St. John's House was placed under the direction of the All Saints Sisterhood, which had been founded in 1851. Eventually, this Order provided training in midwifery as well as in nursing, and took over the latter service in several London hospitals.

Similar Anglican groups were organized in the United States. The first of these, the Sisters of the Holy Communion, appeared in 1845 and provided the nursing at St. Luke's Hospital in New York City. These American sisterhoods were similar in spirit to their English counterparts; and both, indeed, had much in common with Catholic orders devoted to the same purpose. The Anglican groups tended to be somewhat more free from Church discipline, but all held that their work was primarily of a religious nature.

Somewhat analogous developments occurred in Protestant areas in Germany and in Holland, where there was a revived interest in the early Christian ideal of the Deaconess. Such dedicated persons had been appointed from time to time since the Reformation, and in certain centers elaborate programs had been set up for aiding the poor. Schools, orphanages, and hospitals had been established under Church auspices. A new impetus was given to this tradition when

Theodor Fliedner became pastor at Kaiserswerth on the Rhine in 1822.

Fliedner both influenced and was influenced by English humanitarians. Seeking funds for his struggling parish, he visited England and was impressed by the social work which the Quaker idealist Elizabeth Fry was carrying on in London prisons. Fliedner and his wife, Frederike Münster, thereupon set up a small refuge for discharged prisoners at Kaiserswerth. Becoming concerned about the general lot of the poor, they added an orphanage, a normal school, and a small hospital to their parochial program (1835–1842).

In 1836 the first Deaconess was brought into the hospital and others followed. By 1842 the institution had grown to one of over 200 beds, and the Deaconesses were asked to nurse in the municipal hospital of a neighboring city. Subsequently, after the death of his first wife, Pastor Fliedner married Caroline Bertheau; and the latter, who had been superintendent of a surgical ward in Hamburg, took over the training of nurses. Distinctions were made between Probationers and those accepted as Deaconesses, and the course was lengthened.

Meantime, Fliedner sent out groups of Deaconesses to the Near East and one was also established at Pittsburgh in this country. These units devoted themselves to various good works; and where they served in hospitals, they maintained the type of nursing training which had been received at the "Motherhouse" in Kaiserswerth. Deaconesses were not bound by vows, however, and could leave the service if they so wished.

The chief achievement of Anglican Sisters and of German Deaconesses was to introduce superior women into at least a few of the hospitals of Protestant countries. This, in itself, improved the character of nursing care in such institutions and set an example which led to further attempts in this direction. Being relatively free, moreover, these groups—especially St. John's House and the Motherhouse at Kaiserswerth—provided more formal hospital training than had hitherto been customary among nursing orders.

Early Schools of Nursing

The fact remains that Anglican Sisters and German Deaconesses, like the Catholic orders, maintained the tradition of Church-directed nursing services. Other tendencies, however, were beginning to manifest themselves in Protestant countries. The inherited opposition to religious orders probably limited the expansion of nursing sisterhoods in Great Britain and in the early United States; and sometimes this attitude found overt expression.

Rather striking, for example, was the program set up in the Swiss city of Lausanne in 1859. Here the Comtesse Agénor de Gasparin founded and endowed a training school for nurses. This was termed "evangelical" as an indication of Christian attitudes, but it was not in any sense the motherhouse of an order. The students, moreover, had to be more than pious; they received regular instruction from physicians as well as ward experience. Upon graduation, they were to serve as superior lay nurses on a salaried basis. This school, known as "La Source," prospered during ensuing decades.

One could observe at Lausanne the convergence of two relatively new influences upon nursing; that is, the increasing secularization of the age, and the realization that current medical developments called for the specific medical instruction of future nurses.

La Source, as a matter of fact, was not the first training center which responded to these influences. The example of a formal school for lay nurses, introduced at Mannheim by Franz May as early as the 1780's, was followed in other German cities during the next half century. In 1832, for example, such a school was set up in connection with certain Berlin hospitals. Here both men and women were accepted as candidates if they were literate and could demonstrate good character. Formal instruction in all aspects of nursing was provided by a physician for a period of four months; and the students also spent two months under supervision as probationary nurses in a local hospital (the Charité). Finally, upon passing an examination, they were certified as trained nurses.

Although these arrangements were elementary by modern standards, they foreshadowed many of the features of present-day education. Note, also, that the Berlin school originated with physicians and hospital officials, rather than with individual humanitarians. This, in itself, suggests that at least a few clinicians desired better nursing care as part of their *medical* program.

The next forward step in nursing, however, was to be made in England rather than in Germany. Like most things English, at the time, this was inspired by voluntary rather than by official humanitarianism. But by the mid-century, when this occurred, idealism was by no means restricted to church circles; and secular reformers were more apt than were religious orders to be aware of the medical implications of nursing. The epic of Florence Nightingale must be recalled against this background, since the promise of a medically-trained, lay nursing profession was becoming apparent to some observers by 1850.

Florence Nightingale's Contributions to Nursing and Hospital Administration

Florence Nightingale was born in Florence, Italy in 1820, and derived her given name from that city. Her parents were a wealthy English couple, whose travels on the Continent provided their daughter with a cosmopolitan background. She enjoyed other advantages, such as a classical education and influential connections. Social life as such, however, made no appeal to her. Deeply religious by nature, she was keenly aware of human misery all about her and early decided that the best way to serve God was by helping mankind.

Miss Nightingale was by no means a sentimental reformer. She was philosophically inclined but also quite realistic, and she admired those who applied religious principles to society more than those who merely contemplated them. Although inspired by Christian idealism, this woman's approach was secular in the sense that she represented no particular Church and sought to enlist all of good will in helping their fellow men. She thus reflected, but in most unusual measure, the passion for social reform which was characteristic of her time.

It was not easy for Florence Nightingale to break away from the fashionable life of English country houses. The respectable thing for a young lady, after Continental tours and presentation at Court, was to remain at home and marry. Conversely, it was unheard of for a "genteel female" to take any position in the work-a-day world. Only religious orders offered respectability outside the home, and it is not strange that Miss Nightingale felt drawn toward those which served so useful a purpose as nursing. At the age of twenty-five she was already dreaming of providing a small house for the sick poor, where "something like a Protestant Sisterhood, without vows, for women of educated feelings, might be established."[43] But the family put a stop to this; they were "terrified" at the thought of their daughter doing anything so menial and revolting as to serve in a hospital.

Miss Nightingale did not waver in intent, but bided her time during further trips abroad. While in Rome in 1847, she came to know and admire the training received in Catholic sisterhoods; and two years later, she visited Pastor Fliedner's center at Kaiserswerth. This so impressed her that she returned for three months' residence in 1851. Although she did not think well of the hospital training there, she was greatly impressed by the spirit of the Fliedners and their Deaconesses. In 1852 and '53 she sought to secure nursing training in Catholic institutions in Ireland and in France, but illness and other circumstances prevented. Finally, in '53, she became superintendent of an "Establishment for gentlewomen during Illness" in London.

The Nightingale family accepted this arrangement with as much grace as was possible and Florence was provided with an allowance which stood her in good stead thereafter. She had, at this time, received little formal training in nursing; but she had carefully observed hospitals in four countries and was unusually well-informed on the whole subject. She remained a year at the London institution, gaining experience and revealing marked administrative ability. She had her plans, and displayed skill and determination in persuading the board and the physicians to carry them out.

Two circumstances were in her favor. Since she needed no salary, she could talk to the "society" women on the board on their own terms. Moreover, although most upper-class people still disapproved of careers for women, the feminist movement had been stirring for some time and "liberal" thinkers were becoming open-minded about the issue. This was particularly true in Great Britain and in the United States; in the latter, for example, a medical school for women had been founded in 1850. Although Miss Nightingale disdained the more extreme feminists, she was seriously interested in greater opportunities for her sex and became well known to influential British leaders who shared this attitude.

The small London institution, of course, offered little beyond a

[43] Quoted in Sr. Edward Cook, *Life of Florence Nightingale*, I, The Macmillan Co. (New York, 1942), 44.

chance to acquire experience. How Miss Nightingale's great opportunity came suddenly and unexpectedly in 1854 has been repeatedly told and has become the epic of modern nursing. In that year, Great Britain, France, and Turkey declared war on Russia in order to prevent the latter from seizing Constantinople (Istanbul). And in that year, the allied forces invaded the Crimea area in southern Russia and suffered heavy losses in the opening battles. British hospital facilities for their wounded were almost nonexistent. A special correspondent at the front (such service was just beginning) wrote the London *Times* that the barracks used as hospitals contained neither surgeons, nurses, nor the "commonest appliances of a workhouse sick ward." Since the French army had nursing Sisters in their wards, the correspondent added the startling question, "Why have we no Sisters of Charity?"

The response to this report was dramatic, for few could resist an appeal which combined patriotism and humane feeling. No sick or wounded men should be so neglected, least of all those who were fighting for their Queen. Florence Nightingale wrote at once to Sydney Herbert, an old friend who was then "Secretary at War" in the British Government, and offered to take a group of nurses out to the hospital based at Scutari in Turkey. Her letter crossed with one from Mr. Herbert, making just this request of her.

The Secretary at War knew that it was revolutionary to propose sending decent women into army hospitals—of all places! Religious orders commanded respect even among troops but it was doubted if lay women could do so.[44] But Mr. Herbert had confidence in Florence Nightingale as the one person who could both save the Scutarian situation and establish the reputation of good nursing for all time to come.

Miss Nightingale promptly accepted the invitation and was appointed Superintendent of Army Nurses in Turkey under the War Office. Gathering a group of thirty-eight nurses, which included Catholic and Anglican Sisters as well as lay women, she arrived at Scutari on November 4, 1854. Popular sympathy had provided her with a fund which eventually reached £7,000 (more than $100,000 in today's

[44] Distrust on this score persisted in Latin Europe long after it was overcome in English-speaking countries. As late as World War I (1918), French opinion is said to have been shocked by the appearance of respectable American or British women who served in Salvation Army huts near the front.

currency), and she had had the foresight to purchase some supplies with this on the way out.

Pages could be written on the chaos which she found at the Scutari barracks. Buildings were unsanitary and vermin infested, no decent food was available, and only straw and canvas sheets could be had for bedding. A few overworked surgeons and some undisciplined orderlies provided all the medical attention which could be secured. The small group of nurses had not only to face this chaos, but also the opposition of medical officers who opposed any reform as a criticism of their own incompetence.

Miss Nightingale's first task was to clean up the buildings and secure supplies. This was done, at first, largely through the use of her own funds. She displayed a mastery of detail and gradually introduced order into the vast shambles, which soon included four miles of beds separated from one another only by inches. Something like humane nursing was provided, as more nurses were sent out. Florence Nightingale herself was most compassionate, and this "Lady with a lamp" became the object of true devotion among the ill and wounded.

Meanwhile, she had to contend with official inertia and disapproval. Old medical officers would have resented the intrusion of any woman, but they particularly disliked the interference of this one whom they nicknamed "the Bird." For what *they* saw was not compassion but an aggressive, almost domineering demand for reform. Miss Nightingale was technically under the supervision of the Medical Department, and she always insisted on a strict obedience to orders— including her own. But she had powerful friends in London and much popular support, and with the use of such backing she usually secured her own way.

Eventually, she extended her control to hospitals in the Crimea, where she became seriously ill in the process. Once the most basic improvements had been made in the hospitals at both Scutari and the Crimea, she found time for other innovations which have since become routine. To divert convalescents from drunkenness and other demoralizing conditions, for example, she set up recreation huts and even persuaded many men to send money home to their families.

The Superintendent worked night and day and drove others in like manner, but there was no doubting the results. The death rates in army hospitals declined dramatically, the patients were touchingly grateful, and all England applauded. Queen Victoria was impressed and praised this heroic Englishwoman as an ornament to her sex.

When Florence Nightingale returned to England in 1856, she was already a legend. Popular subscriptions were gathered in her name, which amounted eventually to £44,000. It was expected that she would give this to some good cause, but most people probably assumed that her own work was over. She was known to be ill and had she not done enough? But the object of all this adoration had only begun. She did not recover health for some years, and the terrible memories of Scutari continued to haunt her. But this, in itself, doubtless drove her on to further efforts. As she wrote in 1856: "I stand at the altar of the murdered men, and, while I live, I fight their cause."[45]

One need not review here all the "causes" to which Miss Nightingale gave herself over the ensuing three decades. During the late 1850's she attained, through her general influence and also through direct contacts with British officials, a sweeping reform of the Medical Department of the British Army. She actually secured the founding of an Army Medical School. During the 1860's, again, she exercised a somewhat similar influence over British administration in India. Just because she was a woman, she could not assume official, political position, but she became literally a power behind the throne. And she always directed this power in the direction of humane reform.

Of most immediate interest were her contributions to nursing and to hospital administration. Before tracing this theme, however, a final word may be said about Florence Nightingale herself. She played such a commanding and dramatic role in introducing modern nursing, that her personality has been interpreted in varying ways in an effort to explain her achievements. Long praised as the great heroine of the nineteenth century, she has in recent decades also been subjected to adverse criticism. This shift in itself reflects the changing temper of different eras—from the romantic enthusiasms of Victorian days to the critical, psychological insights of the present century.

Miss Nightingale spent most of her long life after 1856 as a semi-invalid (she lived until 1910), and this fact has suggested to some that she had a neurotic personality, or that she pleaded illness because it provided seclusion, or that she found it afforded a dramatic

[45] Cook, *Florence Nightingale*, 318.

setting. More serious is the indictment that she was a religious fanatic, whose intense drive forced herself and those she used beyond all natural endurance. One biographer implies, for example, that she drove Sydney Herbert to his death—and only then sanctified him as her "master."[46]

There is undoubtedly evidence that Miss Nightingale's personality had its unpleasant side. She was demanding and persistent, and often sharp with those who faltered in following her. She desired power and was not always an easy person to work with. But one should also recall what she had been through, and for what purposes she desired power.

Last but not least, one may well inquire: What sort of woman *could* get results on a public scale in the mid-nineteenth century? Surely, the conventionally gracious lady would have had little chance against the obstacles of massive conservatism. There must have been a sort of natural selection, as reformers, of women who *were* aggressive and therefore not the most pleasant of individuals. One notices similar traits in other feminine reformers between 1850 and 1900—it took that kind! Once the reforms were accomplished, the gracious ladies could again come forward.

In any case, Florence Nightingale's contributions to nursing and to hospital administration stand on their own merits. In considering these, one can take up for the first time a series of developments which led directly into modern nursing.

The Nightingale Plan for Nursing Education

The Superintendent of Army Nurses had found it most difficult to secure qualified women for her hospital service in Scutari. The entire experience had impressed on her the need for adequate training for such service, on a scale which could not be met by the small English sisterhoods.

It was not enough, in her view, to just secure better women—desirable as this was in itself. The best of women would be useless if ignorant. Although this statement now seems self-evident, one must recall that any good woman was then supposed to have an intuitive, humane instinct for nursing. Miss Nightingale was not the first to

---

[46] [G.] Lytton Strachey, in *Eminent Victorians*, G. P. Putnam's Sons, New York, 1918, 185 ff.

say that knowledge as well as character was essential in this work, but she was the first to say it so effectively that entire nations took heed. As she pointed out, no one claimed that good intentions alone could qualify a man to be a physician. By the same token, as demands on nurses became more complex, no one should think a woman fit to be a nurse merely because she was a nice person.

Since Miss Nightingale's opinions were well known, it was first assumed that she might direct a new school of nursing which could serve as a model of its kind. When her illness prevented this, the trustees of the Nightingale Fund investigated several London hospitals where the proposed school might be established. Arrangements were finally completed with St. Thomas's Hospital, an institution which had many advantages for the purpose. The medical director was sympathetic; and the Matron, Mrs. Wardroper, had already made improvements in the nursing staff. With Florence Nightingale's full approval, the School of Nursing was therefore set up in St. Thomas's and Mrs. Wardroper took charge under her old title. The first students, fifteen in number, were admitted in June, 1860.

Miss Nightingale's plan, as unfolded in the School, involved two innovations. The first was that the Fund provided an endowment which enabled the School to pay its own way. There was no financial obligation to St. Thomas's and the School could therefore place educational values above routine nursing needs of the Hospital. This advantage was lost in many, subsequent nursing schools, which were organized by hospitals with a view to securing free or low-price probationers to serve in their wards. The original, St. Thomas emphasis on education, however, has been revived in nursing schools in recent decades.

The second innovation also could be insisted upon because the St. Thomas School paid its own way. Hitherto, as noted, lay nurses had been under the authority of men as hospital directors or medical staff members, and the consequent treatment of the nurses as servants had been one of the chief obstacles to morale among the nursing personnel. Florence Nightingale had directed her nurses at Scutari within an all-feminine organization, and this arrangement was now adopted in the new School. Here and in other schools which followed, the fact that women were in charge assured some improvement in status for the student group.

The students at St. Thomas' received a year's training which included instruction from the Matron, the ward "Sisters" (head nurses), and the physicians. They were then added to the nursing staff of the Hospital for two years, where they gained experience under supervision. Remaining as probationers (student nurses) throughout this period, most were paid modest salaries from the endowment; while others, intended later to fill higher positions, themselves paid tuition during the first year.

This distinction between ordinary probationers and "lady nurses" reflected British class consciousness. The former group continued to be drawn from relatively uneducated levels, and something of the old servant tradition still clung to them. The gentlewomen who paid their own way, on the other hand, were relieved of some of the drudgery in training and were expected to become matrons in the future. Questionable as this distinction may now seem, it probably made it easier for British society of the 1860's to accept the St. Thomas program.

After completing two years in the wards, the probationers became full-fledged "Sisters" (nurses) and continued to "live in" at the hospital unless called to another institution or given other assignments. Upon completion of any special work, they returned to the hospital as their permanent home. In this arrangement, one can again observe the persistence of older forms; in this case, of the idea of the "mother house" and of a semi-enclosed life. Nightingale nurses were not yet independent women, free to seek their own opportunities and to come and go as they pleased. Nursing, Miss Nightingale was convinced, was not a profession but rather a "calling."

The same ideal was maintained by Mrs. Wardroper at St. Thomas'. She continued to serve there as Matron until 1887, and as such had full control over the school, over all nursing in the hospital, and even over the kitchen and domestic staff. A strict disciplinarian, she was responsible only to the hospital board. Something of her authority, however, was passed on to the ward Sisters (head nurses) who required implicit obedience from other nurses and probationers, and who carried on most of the practical instruction.

Such a regime would be resented by most lay nurses today, but severe discipline and moral oversight of nurses seemed natural enough in the 1860's. The system also had practical advantages at the time.

No one had yet proved that lay women could make as good or even better nurses than the religious Sisters, and any failure or scandal at the start would have retarded the whole effort. St. Thomas' had to set an example.

The first result of this example was that Nightingale nurses were in demand at other hospitals as soon as they were available. The upper-class women at St. Thomas' had been "trained to train"; and, whenever a hospital appealed to Miss Nightingale for aid, she would arrange to have one or more of these persons go out to found a new nursing school. A series of such institutions was founded in this way in London, in other British cities, and in those of the Dominions. Wherever established, these hospital schools largely reproduced the features of "the Nightingale system" as just described.

The proliferation of training schools provided trained nurses who gradually replaced the old personnel. The process, of course, did not happen all at once. "Nightingale nurses" naturally expected better accommodations and salary than had the older attendants, and some hospitals could not at first meet these requirements. But recognition of the need for higher standards eventually forced readjustments, and most British and Dominion hospitals were supplied with trained, lay nurses by the end of the century.

The Sanitary Ideal and Modern Nursing

For some three decades after 1860 Miss Nightingale, amidst all her other activities, continued to guide and watch over the expansion of nursing education. This she did not only by personal contacts but through her writings as well, and the influence of the latter reached far beyond England. For the sake of clarity, one may distinguish between the guidance she provided concerning the ideals of nursing, on the one hand, and its methods on the other.

As already mentioned, Florence Nightingale maintained that nursing was a "calling"; her "Sisters" must be devoted to a cause. The moral values of this ideal were beyond question, but it tended to inhibit the development of such professional outlooks as were taken for granted among other lay groups. Yet, as the number of trained nurses grew, some of them became conscious of common interests which transcended loyalty to their particular schools. They had before them the example of professional societies among physicians and other trained personnel, and it seemed logical enough that nurses also should organize in their own interest.

Out of this conflict in ideals emerged the "Nurses Battle" of 1886–1893. In the first of these years, a group of nurses founded the British Nurses Association and announced their desire to set up a General Register of Nurses. Such a Register had been provided by Parliament for physicians in the 1850's, and included all those who had received proper education and could meet certain tests. Since this system had protected the public against unqualified medical practitioners, why could not an analogous Register for nurses serve a similar function in their field? So, at least, reasoned its proponents.

Plausible as this idea now appears, it seemed at the time to threaten the most cherished values of the St. Thomas tradition. National registration, declared Miss Nightingale, would include the worst as well as the best nurses—it could make no such distinctions as could the individual schools. Worst of all, it could certify only that the nurse had received some training and could tell nothing about her character. And character was of the essence. Or, as she put it, ". . . nurses cannot be registered and examined any more than mothers."[47] What could a Register tell of the moral environment in the nursing school, or of the nurse's "sense of duty and love of the calling?"

Miss Nightingale apparently sensed that nursing was getting beyond the bounds of the idealistic, semi-enclosed group which she had ever in mind. If an organized profession emerged, it could no longer be controlled by her type of school and it would doubtless exhibit a "mercantile spirit" devoted to material things—such as "forcing up wages." Nursing, she held, might then gain the world but would lose its own soul.

The outcome, after several years of controversy, was that the Queen granted the Association a royal charter in 1893 and permitted it to maintain a list of such nurses as wished to appear therein. But the Association was given no exclusive right to register nurses nor any control over nursing education. The Association had meantime founded its own journal, *Nursing Record,* and through this claimed a victory in principle. In reality, the settlement seems to have been a compromise.

[47] Cook, *Florence Nightingale*, II, 359.

This compromise, nevertheless, represented another step away from a religious orientation toward a professional outlook. Nurses' societies and journals had come to stay. In this respect Miss Nightingale, although usually viewed as the founder of modern nursing, may also be viewed as a transitional figure. She secularized the service in some measure but never gave up the religious ideal inherited from the nursing orders.

With regard to Miss Nightingale's influence on nursing methods, one again observes this pattern of contributions which were limited by the outlook of her formative years. She displayed much insight, derived from experience, into the detailed niceties of nursing —how to dress, walk, talk, and the like. These things were important. But, in more general matters, her whole program was inspired by the enthusiasm for sanitary reform which was at its height in the 1850's. Whereas most sanitarians pursued this interest in the public health field, Florence Nightingale applied it to hospitals and nursing. She was, then, one of the great sanitarians, albeit of a specialized sort.

Hospitals, she held, should be built on the pavilion plan so as to assure fresh air and cleanliness. And nurses should provide individual patients with the same fresh air and cleanly surroundings, plus proper beds and clothing, "pure" water, and good food. Like other sanitarians, Miss Nightingale proved the value of such arrangements by resort to vital statistics. The death rates in well-administered hospitals, as compared to those in the old-fashioned types, provided all the justification that she needed.

The limitations of this program were those inherent in the sanitary ideal itself. Sanitarians had reacted against the contagion doctrine of the 1700's, and were convinced that "airs and waters" (the physical environment) largely determined the health of any population. The famous Englishwoman even spoke of "nursing the well," by which she meant providing them with a sanitary regimen. This was laudable and seemed to anticipate recent ideas about promoting "positive health." But, like other sanitarians, she went to extremes in minimizing contagion. She did not even fear that of smallpox—fresh air alone would avert any danger.[48]

Although bacteriologists threw new light on this problem after 1875, Miss Nightingale continued to ridicule the idea of infection.

[48] See, e.g., *Notes on Nursing* (New York, 1860), 32 ff.

She was unable, in a word, to adjust her viewpoint to changing concepts in medical science. Yet she took the science of her own youth most seriously and this proved to have lasting value. The sanitary ideal, within the limits suggested, has continued to be basic in modern nursing.

Other Influences on Nursing Education

Not all of the improvements made in nursing, 1860 to 1900, are to be credited to Miss Nightingale. It has been pointed out that efforts were being made toward this end in other European countries, both before and after 1860. It is almost inconceivable, indeed, that humanitarianism, sanitary reform, and medical progress could have failed to make an impress upon nursing during the last part of the nineteenth century. There is no question, however, that Miss Nightingale's influence publicized this trend, provided a model, and gave the whole movement a marked impetus.

On the European Continent, the Nightingale influence was naturally felt most strongly in Protestant areas—in Holland, the Scandinavian countries, and parts of Germany. In the former, a secular nursing school was provided at Amsterdam in the 1880's, and a Dutch Association for Sick Nursing was set up in 1892. This body developed a strong professional consciousness, sought to improve and unify training standards, and secured legislation which required a state diploma for all nurses.

Similar developments occurred in Norway and Sweden. In the latter, for example, a St. Thomas-trained nurse became matron of a new hospital school at Upsala as early as 1866. Protestant circles also maintained lay training schools at certain cities in Switzerland and in France, as in La Source at Geneva (mentioned above), and in a Nightingale school founded at Bordeaux about 1900. Such centers doubtless set an example of relatively good training standards.

On the Continent, meantime, a further stimulus for nursing reform appeared in the international Red Cross organization. The movement to found such a body grew, as had Miss Nightingale's efforts, out of sympathy for the sufferings of sick and wounded soldiers. A Swiss observer, Jean Henri Dunant, happened to be present at the battle of Solferino in Italy in 1859, when the French and Italians were victorious in a war against the Austrians. He was depressed by the lack of medical services; and appealed subsequently to various European governments to set up an international organization which could provide disciplined, volunteer nursing aid on battlefields.

In 1863, by the "Convention of Geneva," twelve governments founded the international Red Cross—so called because of its emblem. National, member societies were set up, which were to prepare during peace for offering their services during war. In case of hostilities, the personnel of these societies were to be placed under military discipline and were to display distinctive insignia in the field. Each government agreed to honor Red Cross nurses as noncombatants, and to respect their hospitals and other facilities. Red Cross societies in neutral countries, moreover, were to be permitted to give humanitarian services to belligerents on either side.

Within two years after 1863, thirteen national Red Cross societies had been formed, each a member of the international organization. The rapidity of these developments can be ascribed partly to patriotic sympathy for the wounded of one's own country, but it should not be overlooked that a broader, humane ideal was also involved.

The first thought had been that a Red Cross society would provide men and women volunteers with elementary training (as in "first aid") which would enable them to give emergency service during war. But the international Red Cross was caught up in the whole trend toward better nursing, and so decided at its 1869 conference that volunteer workers should receive regular training and pass examinations. This decision involved the national societies in a program of training nurses, and that in turn led them to acquire their own hospitals and schools.

The national societies soon expanded their interests to include aid in special disasters (earthquakes, fires) as well as in war, and eventually acquired a concern about public health in general. But between 1865 and 1900, they were most active in Europe in hospital and nursing work—in civilian as well as in the military services. Although the training received by Red Cross nurses continued to be elementary in some countries, in others it took on the form of regular nursing schools. In Russia, for example, military hospitals were placed at the disposal of the Red Cross, and three-year training courses were set up therein. By 1897, four such schools had trained nearly 3,000 nurses.

In Western Europe, meantime, a complicated pattern of nursing education was emerging. Catholic and Protestant sisterhoods continued to operate traditional programs but introduced into these extended educational requirements. Side by side with these were Red Cross hospitals and schools, which were lay in character but which tended to retain the "mother house" system which was so generally accepted in these countries. And here and there, as noted, were Nightingale training schools directed by English-trained matrons.

The balance of these different systems is suggested by the situation in Germany, where religious sisterhoods, the Red Cross, and secular training schools were all in operation. By 1907, for example, a total of 75,000 women nurses was recorded. Of these, 26,000 were Catholic Sisters, 12,000 were Protestant Deaconesses, and some 4,000 were Red Cross nurses. Of the remainder, about 3,000 belonged to a professional nursing association.

Continental training schools exhibited no such uniformity in organization or standards as did the Nightingale system. Schools for Catholic sisterhoods were usually connected with hospitals, but some of those maintained by Deaconesses or by the Red Cross were not. In any case, authority over ward nursing and over the school was not concentrated in one matron as in England, but was divided between hospital officials (committees, chaplains, directors) on the one hand, and a "Superior" of the school on the other. But the latter was usually responsible herself to the hospital authorities, unless the school was quite independent. Practical instruction in the wards was given, in the hospital schools, by Ward Sisters (head nurses) as in England.

Among the sisterhoods and in some of the Red Cross schools, the "motherhouse" tradition carried on. The Sisters "lived in" at the hospital or in a special home, received no salary, and were maintained for life. Independent nursing schools, however, sometimes housed their own students. Again, in secular training programs inspired by British example, students lived in nursing homes under a "Home Sister" and were free agents after graduation.

Generally speaking, one may say that the religious orientation of nursing continued to prevail in Catholic lands, that secular nursing became common in English-speaking countries, and that both these outlooks flourished in Holland, Germany, and Scandinavia. Red Cross institutions reflected whatever type of nursing existed in a given country.

The sisterhoods, whether Catholic or Protestant, retained the great merit of devotion to service and the dignity associated therewith. This was the spirit which Florence Nightingale hoped to retain even within lay nursing. But as such nursing became more secular, it naturally sought to attain professional recognition in the place of religious sanctions. And such recognition, in the nature of the case, involved technical fitness as well as moral values. Hence it was often secular nursing which first responded, as in England, to the need for some medical training of nurses.

Too sharp a line should not be drawn, however, between religious and secular institutions in this field. There were some sisterhoods which responded to the need for medical training, and some secular schools which did not. It should also be remembered that secular nurses, of whatever faith, continued to be guided as individuals by their own religious convictions.

On the whole, and under whatever forms, the standards of nursing rose throughout most parts of Europe between 1860 and 1900. Formal training was more and more insisted upon, and organized, lay nursing became increasingly respectable. This latter trend involved another extension of opportunities for women in general; and it was no accident that lay nursing advanced most rapidly in just those lands, such as Great Britain, Holland, and Scandinavia, where the whole social position of women was a favorable one.

It need hardly be added that, in most countries, the great majority of nursing students after 1860 were women; since the sisterhoods as well as lay personnel took over the care of male wards. "Male nurses," who were hardly distinguishable from orderlies, continued to outnumber women in military services, but this was a vestige of the old order. By the end of the century, nursing was generally viewed as a woman's vocation, and difficulties were experienced in finding such men nurses as were actually needed.

European nursing standards gradually extended into other parts of the world, in so far as Western influences prevailed. Latin America responded to French and Spanish institutions, India to the English, and Japan to general Western examples. Most striking progress, however, was made in the United States and it is this story which particularly concerns us here.

British Influences on American Nursing

Early hospitals in the English American Colonies had naturally followed the patterns of the mother country. Almshouses, such as those set up in Boston, New York and Philadelphia, had included infirmaries where the sick poor were attended by other inmates. These were not hospitals in the modern sense, and only later did their infirmaries evolve into separate, municipal hospitals. Not until 1848, for example, did Bellevue in New York emerge as an institution devoted entirely to the care of the sick.

The nursing in these institutions—if it could be called that—was as crude and indifferent as anything reported in London in the same period. Particularly revolting was the treatment of the insane, and the demoralization of pauper "nurses" whenever epidemics appeared. During an outbreak of cholera in 1832, for example, the attendants at the Philadelphia General ("Old Blockley") were found to be in a state of continuous intoxication; and the situation was temporarily saved only by bringing in Catholic Sisters of Charity.

Meantime, as noted earlier, voluntary hospitals modeled on those of London had been founded in the chief cities—beginning with the Pennsylvania in Philadelphia (1751) and the New York Hospital (1771). These were the first hospitals in the full sense of the term. They were managed by boards composed of "the best people," possessed endowments, and cared for a few private patients; hence they could employ nursing attendants and sought "experienced and trustworthy persons" for such service. Little is known about this personnel, for the hospital authorities did not deem them worthy of comment. But one may assume that they were of a better sort than were the inmates of almshouses, albeit quite untrained save by experience.

The first effort made to educate women in medical services in this country seems to have been that of Dr. William Shippen of Philadelphia, who in 1762 provided lectures in obstetrics to midwives as well as to medical students. In 1798 Dr. Valentine Seaman, of the New York Hospital, also gave lectures to midwives and addressed himself at the same time to nurses. Seaman, like Shippen, assumed that most obstetrical practice would remain in the hands of women and that they should be educated accordingly. This was not the outcome in the United States, though it was in many parts of Europe.

In any case, Dr. Seaman does not seem to have made a sharp distinction between midwifery and nursing; and his lectures on anatomy, physiology, and child care were probably heard by some of the ward attendants. These talks did not constitute a nursing school, nor did they involve such a general program as Dr. May and other German professors advocated in the 1790's. But they did indicate a dawning realization that nurses needed some sort of training.

A generation later in Philadelphia, then the chief medical center of the country, another effort was made to provide trained women for obstetrical nursing. This took the form of a Nurse Society, suggested by Dr. Joseph Warrington of the Philadelphia Dispensary and composed of philanthropic Quaker ladies. Women were recruited, given talks by Dr. Warrington, certified after some practice, and sent out to nurse under supervision in various city districts. The nurses were paid by the Society, and in 1850 were established in a Home and School as their permanent headquarters. It was hoped that general nursing service could be provided for the poor in this way, though actually the only calls received were for obstetrical cases.

Here one observes a closer approach to a lay school than had yet appeared in this country, though the brief training and limited service involved did not constitute a nursing school in the modern sense. Times were changing, of course, by 1850. Certain nursing orders, as noted, had been founded or introduced into the United States by this year; and the Churches—Catholic, Protestant, and Jewish—were beginning to establish their own hospitals.

The feminist movement, moreover, was gaining public attention despite much criticism and ridicule. While poor women had partly replaced men as workers in the textile mills, "advanced women" were demanding the right to vote and to enter the professions. Must "woman's sphere" remain entirely restricted to the home?

In 1850 the Woman's Medical College was established in Philadelphia; and during the next two decades, similar colleges and "women's hospitals" were founded in other seaboard cities. One of the chief arguments advanced in defense of these institutions was that women were entitled to medical care by their own sex, especially in obstetric and gynecologic services. This note was sounded more often in the United States than in Europe, and may have expressed some second thoughts about the loss of midwives. It may also explain the fact that early American concern about better nursing usually related to obstetrical care.

Male obstetricians, however, were not impressed, and insisted that women were not mentally qualified for medical practice. An outstanding authority in Philadelphia praised the genteel female for "her beauty and her grace" but added flatly that, "She has a head almost too small for intellect but just big enough for love."[49] He did not say whether this cranium was big enough for trained nursing, but presumably never even thought of such a program.

The fact that women physicians appeared in the United States somewhat earlier than they did in Europe, played a part in promoting the improvement of American nursing. These women were conscious reformers, they were on trial, and they were anxious that their hospitals should be above reproach. Hence they were concerned about nursing, as well as medical practice, from the start. Thus, the Woman's Hospital—connected with the Woman's Medical College in Philadelphia—opened a nursing school in 1861 and received the first pupils there two years later.

Similar developments were under way in Boston. In 1860 Dr. Marie Zakrzewska, who was appointed professor of obstetrics at the New England Female [Medical] College there, began training nurses. Few women applied, but six were trained over the next two years. The concept of trained, lay hospital service was still a novel one and throughout the 1860's it was difficult to find candidates. But Dr. Zakrzewska took the idea with her to the New England Hospital for Women and Children at nearby Roxbury, and there she trained some thirty nurses during the decade following 1862. These women gave their services in the Hospital for six months in exchange for instruction and were then considered qualified for private service.

Up to this point, no one in the United States seems to have urged that superior women should be "trained to train"; that is, prepared to go out and direct other programs. Hence no group of schools grew up here in the 1860's, like the one which branched out from St. Thomas' in London during that decade.

The delay in following Miss Nightingale's ideas, which were now

49 C. D. Meigs, *Females and Their Diseases*, Philadelphia, 1848, Introduction.

well known in America, can be largely ascribed to the outbreak of the Civil War. This conflict, as did the Crimean War, aroused interest in nursing; but it was such a catastrophe that most activities along this line were diverted into the military services.

When the Civil War began, numerous untrained women volunteered as nurses; and a few individualists like Clara Barton continued to serve independently throughout the struggle. Some order had to be brought into such service, however, and the War Department of the Union Government appointed Dorothea Dix[50] as Superintendent of [Women] Nurses. Miss Dix had already proved an extraordinary leader in improving prisons and founding "insane asylums" in the United States and in parts of Europe. Often compared to John Howard (English prison and hospital reformer), she also had some things in common with Florence Nightingale.

Miss Dix was given authority to appoint and supervise all women nurses in the Union forces, although the latter were directly responsible to the directors of military hospitals in which they served. Like her English counterpart, Miss Dix encountered incompetence and opposition in the Army Medical Corps, and she lacked the powerful official support which had so aided Miss Nightingale. Nevertheless, by dint of determination and careful planning, the Superintendent set up standards for recruitment, secured many volunteers, and made arrangements for the brief training of some of them.

Miss Dix, a Unitarian, never emphasized religious devotion as much as had Florence Nightingale, but she was quite as insistent in requiring good character. Her volunteeers had to be middle-aged, "plain looking," and adorned in more sensible dresses than the conventional hoop-skirts. There was to be no nonsense in her ranks.

Some men also volunteered as nurses, as in the case of the poet Walt Whitman. Male nurses or orderlies outnumbered women in the military wards by two to one. But there is no evidence that the masculine contingent was selected with much care; indeed, many were just assigned from the ranks and received only on-the-spot instruction. Nevertheless, Miss Dix's supervision did something to bring discipline and order into base hospital nursing throughout the Union Army. No such centralized system was arranged on the Confederate side.

[50] Not to be confused with a later, newspaper columnist of some fame.

Before 1861, voluntary societies known as Howard Associations had done something to aid cities visited by epidemics or other disasters, and some enthusiasm for sanitary reform had carried over from England to "the States." Early in the War, groups of earnest women organized similar relief groups, to assure volunteer troops of proper medical supplies, nursing, and other "comforts." Outstanding in such work was Dr. Elizabeth Blackwell, the first woman to take an M.D. in the United States, who gave brief training to some hundred women as nurses for the Union forces.

Out of the relief societies emerged a national Sanitary Commission, which became concerned with the general health of Union troops. This voluntary body, led by distinguished sanitarians, put constant pressure on the Army to reform the disgraceful conditions in many Army camps. In the Civil War, as in the Crimean, far more men died from disease than from wounds, and the improvements introduced by the Commission probably saved more lives than did the services of the Medical Corps.

At the end of the War, there was no such sudden advance in nursing as had followed the Crimean War in England. Miss Dix was unable to repeat the role of Florence Nightingale in this regard for a number of reasons. For one thing, she was already in her sixties and approaching retirement. Nor had nursing been her great love—the care of the insane was always her chief objective. Worn out by work and opposition, her labors were largely finished in 1865.

Real nursing schools therefore did not appear in the United States until the 1870's. When they did come, they were the product of several circumstances. The fact has been noted that certain institutions, particularly those led by women, had been groping toward a training program during the 1850's and '60's. The Civil War had then aroused more public consciousness of the need for sanitary reform in general and for sanitary nursing in particular. Last but not least, European trends had made a cumulative impression by this time. A few Americans had seen nursing education on the Continent; Dr. Zakrzewska, for example, had observed it in The Charité at Berlin. But many more were familiar with Florence Nightingale and her program. Certain persons, Dr. Blackwell for example, knew her intimately; and knowledge of her work and writings was widespread. It was, then, the English example which gave the final impulse necessary to establishing trained nursing in the United States.

In considerable part, this was but another tribute to Miss Nightingale. But it should also be recalled that, quite apart from the merits of the case, the American people were particularly apt to respond to British influences. This was especially true in matters of philanthropy or social reform. Common traditions and language still bound the two countries together, despite political separation. The sanitary drive, for instance, had reached the United States via England. So, too, had the antislavery and women's rights movements; to say nothing of such special societies as the Salvation Army and the Y.M.C.A.

True, the United States also reacted upon Great Britain; but in the nineteenth century the flow of ideas westward across the Atlantic was still greater than the reverse current. All this was perfectly natural under the circumstances. It remained to be seen, however, just how Americans would develop trained nursing, once it had been imported to these shores.

Chapter XIV

American Nursing After 1870:

Problems and Policies

The first American nursing schools, in the modern sense, are said to have been those at Bellevue Hospital in New York City, at the New Haven Hospital, and at the Massachusetts General—all established in 1873. But it will be recalled that the Woman's Hospital in Philadelphia and the New England Hospital for Women and Children had been striving for years to train nurses, and the latter improved its program about this time. One woman who studied there, Linda Richards, is even heralded as "the first trained nurse" in America. Such "firsts," however, rarely have much meaning. In this case, the important fact is that a number of hospitals were founding schools by the early 1870's.

The origins of the Bellevue school illustrates the association of nursing with the larger problems of social welfare. Miss Louisa Schuyler, who had served with the U.S. Sanitary Commission, organized a State Charities Aid Association in New York in 1872. This was a voluntary body concerned with the State's care of paupers, orphans, and the sick; that is, with the conduct of public charity. Their hospital committee inspected the facilities at Bellevue and was startled by its findings. No soap or dishes were available in the wards and "nursing" was done by short-term prisoners. General reform was impossible without a better nursing system. The Association therefore asked the authorities to set up a nurses' training school, presumably on English models.

When the medical board of Bellevue delayed a reply, Dr. Gill Wylie of the staff voluntarily visited English schools for guidance and returned armed with a letter from Florence Nightingale. Mrs. Elizabeth Hobson, Chairman of the Association's hospital committee, then renewed the drive and both the medical board and the Commissioners of Charity finally approved the founding of a school. This was to be under the oversight of the Association's Managers, who contracted to provide the nursing in six wards. Mrs. Hobson announced that they hoped to establish "a college recognized by the State," and would meanwhile appoint a superintendent, provide a comfortable home for nurses, and offer the latter a two-year program. Instruction was given largely by the head nurses in charge of wards, but the medical staff agreed to give some lectures. Head nurses were paid salaries and the students were given small allowances.

The Association inaugurated the School after it had raised a modest fund for the purpose; and Sister Helen Borden of the All Saints sisterhood (Anglican) was made Superintendent. In many respects, Bellevue had the appearance of a Nightingale School. It had modest funds of its own, the Superintendent was not entirely dependent on the medical staff or hospital director, and a good nursing home was provided. Although the students were at first disinclined to accept formal regulations or even to wear a uniform, Sister Helen soon introduced the English type of discipline. This involved a hierarchy of ranks, formal deference to the physicians, and a generally authoritarian atmosphere. But she was an able administrator and convinced a somewhat skeptical medical staff that the School was a real asset to the Hospital. The mortality in its six wards fell well below the earlier rates.

In several respects, however, Bellevue modified the English tradition. Mrs. Hobson rejected the idea of seeking servant probationers, and sought rather students who had had grade school or even academy (high school) education. This was to be the goal of American nurses for decades thereafter. Although some middle-class families still objected to their daughters' becoming nurses, many individuals with this background did enter Bellevue and other early schools.

Mrs. Hobson condemned the notion that any servility was implied when nurses accepted salaries; this was the only way in which lay women could serve. Such women were expected to be religious in outlook but there was to be no sectarianism.

Original instruction was elementary and was crowded into a heavy ward schedule running from 60 to 70 hours a week. Nevertheless, there was a real if limited concern at Bellevue about education. Mrs. Hobson hoped for a program analogous to that of a normal school and opposed any payments to students. Head nurses, functioning as both ward supervisors and instructors, were appointed from among graduates and from other schools. Bellevue graduates also soon went out to direct other schools, much as the St. Thomas's nurses did in England.

No attempt was made to retain the mother house tradition. Although some of the better graduates were appointed as head nurses, the majority went out into private duty. Bellevue set up a registry and an alumnae association, but otherwise the private nurses were "on their own." This was the common outcome in other nursing schools which followed.

Such independence on the part of the individual nurse had advantages, but it also deprived her of security in later years. Wages were not sufficient for savings and there was no mother house to which to return. The lack of personal security continued to worry nurses thereafter, particularly when Americans became more conscious of the whole problem of old age. The advent of federal social security legislation in the 1930's was of some help but did not fully resolve the difficulties.

Some private duty was done in hospitals but the greater part of it was carried on in middle- or upper-class homes. From the nurse's viewpoint, much depended on the character of any given family; but in general the conditions of this work were anything but easy. Many families still thought of a nurse as a semi-servant and expected her to work on a "twenty-four hour schedule." In return for this she received board and low wages—"salary" would be almost too dignified a term under the circumstances.

The poor, of course, could not afford to employ nurses in their homes. But voluntary charitable work was being organized more effectively in the late nineteenth century, and a new vocation of social workers was emerging. Most of these workers were women who shared the ideals of the pioneer nurses and the two groups usually cooperated effectively. As early as 1877, the New York City Mission employed a Bellevue graduate nurse for home nursing in the slums. "Visiting nurses associations" were formed in several cities during the next decade, and these bodies raised funds in order to pay for work of this kind. By 1900 there were twenty such agencies in operation in the larger cities.

The visiting nurse could not live in with a family as did a private duty nurse, and this situation tended to give the former more freedom and even a better status. It was found that much could be done in daily visits, which enabled the nurse to give instruction to both the patient and the family. The very fact that the nurse could not be in the home all the time, made the need for such information more obvious. There were possibilities here for prevention as well as for cure, and these were emphasized when a Boston group adopted the title of Instructive Visiting Nurses Association.

As late as 1900, only about 200 "visiting" or "district" nurses were employed, but demands for them increased as philanthropic activities expanded. Tuberculosis societies, which multiplied after 1904, sent them out to care for poor consumptives—victims of the greatest cause of death in this era. District nurses were likewise employed by agencies which promoted infant welfare. Here and there, industrial plants experimented with nurses who could provide first aid; and boards of education introduced nurses as well as physicians into the elementary schools. The latter program, begun about 1903, was soon followed everywhere. Meantime, visiting nurses became known as "public health nurses," of whom there were about 3,000 by 1912.

Relationships Between Schools of Nursing and Hospitals

One of the basic problems of nursing schools concerned their relationships to the hospitals in which students were trained. St. Thomas' school, one recalls, achieved some independence of the training hospital because it had its own endowment. Its matron had wide powers and was responsible only to the hospital trustees.

The managers representing the Charities Aid Association seem to have hoped for similar status for their Bellevue School, and no one questioned that Sister Helen had full control over the discipline of the nurses. This provided the all-feminine system so dear to Miss

Nightingale's heart, and meantime the managers were inclined to deal directly with the hospital trustees. Mrs. Hobson even hoped to extend feminine influence by having some of her group appointed to the board of trustees. Since women had done much for the hospital, why should they not have a share in its management?

When Sister Helen and the Managers urged the improvement of certain wards, however, the director and medical staff resented this as meddling in *their* affairs. Although Sister Helen finally had her way in this incident, it foreshadowed the attitude of American hospital authorities thereafter. In the case of Bellevue the lines of authority were apparently not clear, since there *was* an outside body which sponsored the nursing school. But thereafter, very few training programs had extra-mural support or funds; and when hospitals founded schools they simply assumed that they would control them.

This trend appeared immediately in the founding of the second nursing school noted, that of the Massachusetts General. Although this school was largely inspired, like Bellevue, by a group of earnest women, the hospital authorities insisted in taking over full direction from the start. The superintendent of the school was made responsible to the director of the hospital, which paid all salaries and maintained a separate matron (housekeeper). The only English administrative tradition which was preserved was the right of the superintendent to select and supervise the nurses.

The third pioneer school, that at the New Haven Hospital, was unusual in owing its start to a group partly made up of men—the General Hospital Society of Connecticut. The Society raised an endowment of $12,000 (about $60,000 in present currency), and here again there may have been some hope of educational autonomy. But the funds were inadequate and the School could scarcely have survived without the idealism and sacrifice of the first women nurses.

The New Haven School illustrates the difficulties which were so common in early programs, until the hospitals took over the schools for their own purposes. There were only four students at first and they acted both as nurses and attendants. They served all day in the wards, sat up at night with typhoid patients, and cooked and distributed meals for thirty patients at a time. As soon as they appeared, the men "nurses" (hitherto in charge of the men's ward) proceeded "to take their ease."

Financing Schools of Nursing

It is hardly surprising that the American public failed to provide funds that would have made nursing schools independent. It required enough readjustment in attitudes, just to recognize that respectable women should go into nursing at all. Nevertheless, lacking funds, nursing schools could be founded only if and when the preexisting hospitals found them useful. This light dawned on hospital authorities when the experience at early schools showed: (1) that better nursing brought down ward mortality, and (2) that the students could provide nursing just in return for "board and keep."

The theory was, of course, that students served in return for education. But the hospitals, always lacking funds themselves, needed the service and therefore tended to let instruction suffer. The hospital in full control of a nursing school need not be particular about entrance requirements, and usually squeezed lectures into odd hours when the ill-prepared students were too tired to listen. Separate classroom buildings were never provided, as for other types of schools, and all theoretical instruction was given in the nurses' homes.

In the better nursing schools like Bellevue, the practical ward instruction was good; but this simply meant that the system had the merits of an apprenticeship. How incongruous this was can be best appreciated by recalling what was happening in the training of physicians at this very time. Medical education was abandoning the apprenticeship of earlier days and focusing all training in classrooms and wards. Moreover, American medical schools retained full independence of the hospitals they used, and even began to set up such institutions (university hospitals) under their own control. Thus, in their relations to hospitals, medical colleges were moving in just the opposite direction from that imposed on nursing schools.

One can readily understand why so many hospitals founded nursing schools. During the 1870's, the number increased slowly because it required time for the pioneer schools to provide superintendents; by 1880 some 15 schools were in existence. But as soon as enough graduate nurses had been "trained to train," hospitals took up this program with avidity. By 1893 some 225 nursing schools had been established, and in 1900 there were no less than 432!

This trend was accelerated by a rapid expansion of hospitals.

There had been only 178 of these institutions in the country in 1873, but by 1909 the number had swelled to over 4,000. Herein one observes the influence of developments in medical science, as noted in a preceding chapter. As the "wonders of modern medicine" began to impress the public, the poor lost some of their old fears and crowded into hospitals. The comfortable classes also sought admission at the guidance of family doctors, especially in connection with "the new surgery."

The expansion of hospitals required additional nurses, many of whom could be supplied from the students in the nursing schools. Eventually, as much of medical practice was transferred from homes to hospitals, there was also need for more graduate nurses in these institutions. This need resulted not only from the sheer number of patients, but also from the fact that the demands made on graduate nurses increased as medicine became more complex. Hence more nurses were needed for a given number of patients than had hitherto been the case.

The rapid proliferation of nursing schools, in response to these circumstances, involved a deterioration in even the apprenticeship aspect of training. Many small hospitals, of less than 100 beds, needed student nurses but were unable to provide diversified ward instruction. Some of them also sent students out on private duty, ostensibly for training but actually in order to collect the fees. And even large institutions set up "short courses," which still further minimized educational elements in their programs.

The great question in all this was not why hospitals founded schools, but rather, why were so many young women willing to enter them? Recall only the long hours, the difficult work, and the subordination to both medical staff and supervisors. And, on the personal side, there was social isolation in even the better nurses' homes.

Yet, after the first few years when only a few students appeared, their numbers mounted along with the multiplication of training programs. By 1898, some 25 of the better schools alone listed 2,500 graduate nurses as members of their alumnae associations; and within another decade the total graduates of all schools approximated 50,000. The number continued to swell thereafter, reaching by the early 1940's about 275,000.

Various factors explain the successful recruiting of nurses during the decades just before and after 1900. In the first place, the conditions of work did not seem as hard then as they would today. Long hours and low pay were typical in farming, business, and industry, as well as in nursing. Some industrial workers, for example, actually "put in" 75 or more hours per week on the night shift as late as 1912.

In the second place, during the earlier decades, the opportunities for women outside the home were still quite limited. Employment in business offices, in telephone exchanges, and the like, became generally available only after 1900. Women had taken over school teaching even as they did nursing, but these two fields and factory work were about all that was open to them. Hence, for a girl who did not wish to be a "factory hand" or a teacher, nursing seemed a promising alternative. This was especially true when economic depressions, as in the 1870's, forced many women to seek jobs.

One should not underestimate, moreover, the role of idealism. It is now common enough to ridicule "tender, loving care"—perhaps because the appeal to idealism was sometimes used to camouflage the exploitation of both teachers and nurses. But there is no question that many of the women who became nurses really wished to help the sick. The Nightingale spirit was by no means lost and one senses it in many accounts of the girls in the better schools. Their rapt devotion often carried them through all the depressing circumstances of training and of its aftermath.

Such idealism was most conspicuous in leading nurses who, after becoming superintendents, struggled to improve the schools and to attain professional status for nurses in general. This story, to which one may now turn, relates to the better schools and to their efforts to maintain a truly educational function. It also involves concomitant attempts to organize nurses throughout the country, both in their own interest and in that of the public welfare.

Early Leaders in Nursing Education

Leadership in American nursing produced no one, outstanding personality like Florence Nightingale, but it fell nevertheless into the hands of some very able figures. This is well illustrated by the activities of three remarkable women who were associated with the founding of the Nursing School at the Johns Hopkins Hospital in 1889—Lavinia L. Dock, Isabel A. Hampton, and M. Adelaide Nutting.

The latter two were Canadians. All three had a background of private schools, possessed scholarly interests, and were attracted to Baltimore by the fame of the new Hopkins Hospital.

Miss Hampton (later Mrs. Hunter Robb) had been trained at Bellevue and was a woman of statuesque beauty as well as of great administrative ability. Her mere appearance before the hospital board was enough to secure her appointment, from among many applicants, as the first Superintendent of the School of Nursing. Miss Dock was made Assistant Superintendent and succeeded Miss Hampton upon the latter's marriage. Miss Nutting, a member of the first class, in turn succeeded Miss Dock.

The Hopkins School of Nursing was unusual, in that provision was made for it in the original planning of the University. When the School opened, the Hospital was in operation but the School of Medicine had not yet begun to function. Hence the former is actually older than the latter. In retrospect, one might think that this situation should have afforded an opportunity for founding an independent, university nursing school. But not even the farsighted Hopkins leaders could envisage such a possibility in 1889. Nevertheless, future medical professors were already available on the Hospital staff and their fame imparted distinction to the whole Hopkins setting. The Misses Hampton, Nutting, and Dock were to play a role, in nursing organizations, which was analogous to that of Doctors Billings, Osler, and Welch within the medical profession.

The Hopkins Nursing School was not distinctive in administration. The Superintendent was responsible to the Hospital Director, and instruction was provided by head nurses and by the medical staff. The Superintendent exercised authority over students and other nurses, and the usual discipline was maintained. In a contemporary note book, Miss Dock remarked on this point:[51]

> The nurse is a soldier. Absolute and unquestioning obedience is the fundamental idea of the military system. . . . There is a necessity for drill in producing quickness, skill and quiet. Criticisms are not accusations. Strictness and exactness produce better nurses.

At Hopkins, as elsewhere, the results of introducing a training

[51] Quoted in Ethel Johns and Blanche Pfefferkorn, *The Johns Hopkins Hospital School of Nurses, 1889–1949*, The Johns Hopkins Press, Baltimore, 1954, p. 76.

program soon overcame any lingering skepticism on the part of the medical staff. And the nursing group undoubtedly benefited by the high caliber of the physicians with whom they were associated. Such men recognized the ability of Miss Hampton and of Miss Dock, and doubtless afforded them more initiative than would have been permitted in most hospitals.

From the beginning, these women sought to improve theoretical instruction as well as practical training. Although elementary, the classes were graded, collateral readings were assigned, and examinations required. In 1896 the program was lengthened from two to three years. In that same year, Miss Nutting—as Superintendent—made an address which was a veritable "Declaration of Rights" for nurses. In this she denounced the exploitation of students, urged that the daily hours of nurses be reduced to eight, and recommended that ward work in the schools be reduced so as to permit more classroom studies. The Hospital Board gave tacit approval to this statement and it provided a creed for the years which followed.

Three years before this, the Hopkins leaders had taken a major part in organizing nurses throughout the country. Envisaging professional status for the field, they realized that this would require associations as well as truly educational programs. The occasion was the Chicago World's Fair of 1893, where Dr. Henry M. Hurd, Director of the Hopkins Hospital, was in charge of a Section of an International Congress of Charities. This Section was devoted to hospitals and nursing.

Arrangements were made by which Miss Hampton and Mrs. Bedford Fenwick, editor of the *British Journal of Nursing,* cooperated in preparing a nursing exhibit. This was good publicity, in a day when Americans—lacking later amusements—flocked to exhibits in droves. Miss Hampton also took the center of the stage by reading another classic letter from Florence Nightingale. British influence thus continued in evidence and Miss Hampton wished to apply it in a specific manner; that is, she planned to follow the example set when the British Nurses Association had been formed in 1886.

Miss Hampton therefore arranged a meeting at Chicago of twenty superintendents of hospital schools, and this group in the following year (1894) organized the "American Society of Superintendents of

Training Schools for Nurses of the United States and Canada."[52] Meantime, Miss Dock and others urged that a general association open to all graduate nurses was likewise needed. After two more years of effort, such a body was founded on the basis of the alumnae groups of some twenty of the better schools. Miss Hampton became the first President of this "Nurses' Associated Alumnae of the United States and Canada" (1896).[53] This body soon represented 26 alumnae groups with a membership of 25,000.

The next logical step toward professional status was to establish a journal. Miss Nutting had urged this as early as the meetings of '93 in Chicago. In 1899 the Nurses' Associated Alumnae set up a journal committee, of which Mary E. P. David (formerly Superintendent of the nursing school at the University of Pennsylvania Hospital) became Chairman. The difficulties faced by this Committee were immense. Was there enough talent available for a publication and, above all, how could necessary funds be secured?

The latter problem was solved by incorporating and issuing stock, which was largely purchased by nurses—poor as many of them were. Miss Sophia F. Palmer, Superintendent of the Rochester (New York) General Hospital School, was then made editor, and the first issue of the *American Journal of Nursing* appeared in 1900.

The *Journal* did not succeed without an initial struggle, since the funds secured were very limited. The only office facilities, in the beginning, are said to have been in Miss Palmer's trunk! Then, too, the majority of private duty nurses—scattered in homes throughout the country—took little interest at the start. Editorial responsibilities fell upon a devoted, volunteer group, which also had to contribute many of the articles. Some of the latter concerned professional questions and aspirations, others related to technical matters. Many of the technical papers now seem dated by their reference to obsolete problems or procedures; for instance, to typhoid nursing, to the care of patients during travel, and to "surgery in the home."

Within a decade, however, the *Journal* was well established. The American Nurses' Association took over all the stock and named the Board, and both the Association and the National League of Nursing Education made the periodical their official organ (1912).

[52] Later shortened to the "National League of Nursing Education" (1912).
[53] Later named the "American Nurses' Association" (1911).

In an early issue, the *Journal* called attention to the rapid increase in the number of public health nurses and to their special needs. Their work was so different from that of ward and private duty, that some special preparation for them was needed in the schools. They also desired an organization of their own which could focus attention on public health nursing in general. The moving spirit in this effort was Lillian D. Wald, founder of the Henry Street Settlement House in Brooklyn, who had first introduced school nursing and who made many other contributions to public welfare.

The two national nursing bodies cooperated; and at their meetings in 1912, various agencies employing public health nurses combined to form the National Organization for Public Health Nursing. A journal was made available to the new body in the preëxisting *Visiting Nurse Quarterly* of the Cleveland Visiting Nurse Association. This publication subsequently became known as *The Public Health Nurse,* and still later as *Public Health Nursing.* After 1912, therefore, three national organizations and two journals were in existence in the nursing field.

Registration of Graduate Nurses

One of the first problems on which the nursing associations focused attention was that of securing legal recognition for graduate nurses. This issue confronts all nascent professional groups and is closely tied in with educational standards. Physicians, for example, had begun to secure state licensing boards even before the American Revolution. Subsequently, medical licensing standards had deteriorated because graduation from a host of poor schools was accepted as granting the right to practice. By 1900, however, physicians had secured a revival of state licensing boards and the beginning of some improvement in medical schools.

The difficulty in nursing, not unlike that in medicine, was that large numbers of people—untrained or poorly trained—were active in practice. When the American Hospital Association[54] looked into the situation, as late as 1913, they found no less than nine types of personnel who served as "nurses." The national associations of nurses made no attempt to limit the right to practice to those who passed

[54] Organized in 1898, and given present name in 1906. It is not as old, therefore, as are the two original nursing organizations.

state examinations, as did physicians, but they did want legislation which would distinguish between graduate and nongraduate personnel. This was clearly desirable in the public interest as well as in their own.

Nursing groups therefore appealed to state legislatures for action. They were not accustomed to such political activity and the way was hard. Nevertheless, their case was a good one and the movement to license and register graduate nurses was becoming world wide. The episode of the "nurses battle" in England, as early as 1886–1893, has been mentioned in this connection. In 1901 the New Zealand legislature passed a Nurses' Registration Act; and similar laws were adopted in five other countries (including several Canadian provinces) between then and 1914.

The first American state to adopt a "nurse practice act" was North Carolina in 1903; and by 1914 some forty other states had followed suit. State examining boards, made up largely of graduate nurses, were appointed. These bodies did not usually examine individuals, as did state medical boards, but set up standards and approved schools which met them. The graduates of such institutions were authorized to use the title "Registered Nurse" (R.N.), in distinction to "practical" or other types of nurses.

In defining standards, the state nursing boards usually specified the minimum number of hours required for theoretical instruction. A few boards required high school graduation for admission to nursing schools, outlined a curriculum, and provided inspection. As implied in all this, the standards were none too high and most boards sought only to reach the level already attained by better schools. Few if any efforts were made to develop truly professional education in the present sense. Nevertheless, the legal status accorded the R.N. was a step toward professional recognition.

How to improve educational standards therefore remained a problem. Administrative control and vested interests usually blocked progress in this direction in hospital schools. Under these circumstances, Miss Hampton envisaged the possibility of securing further education for nurses after they graduated from approved schools. Especially in mind were those who planned to become instructors. This procedure was already employed by school teachers who, after completing normal school work, took further courses in colleges or universities. In 1899 Miss Hampton and others persuaded Dean James E. Russel, of Teachers College, Columbia University, to open his doors to graduate nurses. A course in hospital economics was organized, and in 1907 Miss Nutting was appointed by Columbia as the first full-time professor of nursing in this country.

The device of post-school courses undoubtedly raised the educational horizons of those nurses who "trained to train," and thereby improved national leadership in the field. And the attachment of a nursing program to a university, quite outside of hospital controls, was another forward step. Yet in nursing, as in school teaching, the question would be raised in time: Why should not general college education be provided in the normal and in the nursing schools themselves? Otherwise, it would continue to be an extra obligation, required of practitioners after they had already assumed heavy burdens. Any such question, of course, raised problems concerning the whole program in nursing.

Beginnings of Military Nursing

In the midst of early efforts to advance nursing, this field was subjected to the passing storm of the Spanish-American War (1898–1899). At that time there were still no Army or Navy nursing corps for women, the experience of the Civil War services having been largely forgotten by the military. The American Red Cross had been finally founded under Clara Barton's leadership in 1881, as a constituent of the International body, but had devoted its work chiefly to emergency relief. Hence no Red Cross nurses were available in this country. American battle casualties were small during the Spanish War, but hastily constructed army camps were devastated by typhoid fever and women nurses were desperately needed.

In this emergency, the Nurses' Associated Alumnae offered its services but the Army rejected them. Equally humiliating was the fact that the Army then turned to the Daughters of the American Revolution, with a request that they recruit nurses for the camps. The D.A.R. had funds and influence, and an energetic executive in Dr. Anita N. McGee. She succeeded in working out a program which involved the contract service of some 8,000 volunteer nurses; and this, in effect, represented the beginning of the present Army Nursing Corps.

Meantime, many local and state Red Cross societies became interested in nursing and in volunteer training in first aid. The New York body, for example, set up a Society for the Maintenance of Trained Nurses, which supported and directed their own personnel. More than fifteen years later, when the United States again became involved in war, the American Red Cross secured large funds donated by the American people. And after World War I ended (1918), the organization used these funds to introduce public health nursing in many communities. The American Red Cross, however, did not follow the European example in providing hospitals and nursing schools. This doubtless made easier the subsequent cooperation between the Red Cross and the major nursing societies.

Problems and Trends: 1910–1940

Throughout the three decades following 1910, the chief problems and trends in nursing continued to be those which have now been summarized. World War I established the position of nurses in the military services and promoted respect for the whole guild. Public health nursing, in particular, received increasing recognition with the expansion of public health programs. In infant welfare as well as in schools, the work of such nurses was largely preventive in nature; and they carried this function over even into such home nursing as was supported by the Red Cross, settlement houses, and tuberculosis societies.

During the 1920's a number of "health demonstrations" were carried out in selected communities by the Commonwealth Fund, the Metropolitan Life Insurance Company, and the National Tuberculosis Association, and these demonstrations brought out the central role of public health nurses in community health programs. Thereafter, they were increasingly employed by the official health agencies.

Immediately after World War I, the number of students in nursing schools fell off markedly and considerable alarm was aroused. Some critics blamed the nursing guild itself, and there were demands for quick recruitment and brief training in order to supply the needed numbers. The well-known surgeon, Charles H. Mayo, even published an article entitled: "Wanted, 100,000 Girls for Sub-Nurses." His view, that a two-year training program might be enough, disturbed the nursing organizations which had worked for the three-year curriculum as a standard.

Actually, the decline in the number of students reflected the availability of other opportunities for women, and the relatively discouraging prospects for them in many of the nursing schools. An energetic recruiting program during the 1920's, nevertheless, brought school enrollments up again, and the "White Cap Famine" was forgotten until it would reappear after World War II.

New Developments in Nursing Responsibilities

Something was said, in the preceding chapter, of increasing responsibilities which medical progress imposed on nursing after about 1875. The first generations of "trained" or "graduate" nurses were already expected to perform more medical functions than had been the case with earlier hospital attendants. The former were brought into operating rooms during the 1880's and '90's, and assumed much of the postoperative care. In the medical wards, few procedures yet called for much technical skill but they did require accuracy. Pulse- and temperature-taking, hypodermic injections, and the like were routine by this time. Good judgment might be demanded at any moment, as in deciding whether or not an emergency justified a hurried call on the medical staff.

As scientific advances accelerated thereafter, technical demands on nurses kept pace. By the 1930's and '40's, the whole picture had changed. By this time, surgery included neurologic and even thoracic surgery, and the techniques and instruments involved were far more complex. Internal medicine likewise evolved more complicated diagnostic as well as therapeutic procedures; and busy clinicians tended to turn over some of these activities to graduate nurses and to medical technicians.

This process was a gradual one, but any comparison of nursing procedures in the mid-nineteenth century with those of the past generation will show what a revolution was involved. In 1860, for example, Florence Nightingale had pictured as the nurse's chief functions such simple (though important) matters as providing fresh air, the right food, cleanly rooms and bedding, and generally thoughtful care. Doses were administered as prescribed and the nurse was to report "how the patient was" during intervals between professional calls; but otherwise no strictly medical measures were mentioned.

In contrast, consider the variety and complexity of the graduate nurse's work by the mid-1940's. In an on-the-spot check made at that time in a large teaching hospital—exclusive of operating, obstetrical, and outpatient services—some hundred procedures and treatments were found to be of a more or less technical nature. For example, the nurses took blood pressures, gave gavages, aided in transfusions, and applied suction to surgical wounds, tracheotomies, and chest cavities. They also:[55]

> managed the apparatus for Wangensteen suction, tidal irrigation, and bladder decompression. They irrigated eyes, cecostomies, colostomies [and] draining wounds. . . . They gave colonic irrigations. They did artificial respiration . . . applied sterile compresses and painted lesions. . . . They did catheterizations, sitz baths, and turpentine stupes. They gave insulin and taught the patient or his relatives to give the drug and examine urine. They administered approximately 1,500 medications daily, by mouth or hypodermic. They assisted with lumbar punctures, thoracenteses . . . and phlebotomies.

And so on and on. In all this, the nurse was expected to know each instrument and procedure, to be able to detect toxic reactions or other undesirable developments, to guard the patients against special risks, and to assure the accuracy of all prescriptions. Although the major responsibility of physicians continued to place a sort of ceiling over nursing functions, that ceiling had lifted by the 1940's to a point where nurses were doing more for patients than physicians themselves had done a half-century before.

Nursing organizations responded to such growing demands by efforts to improve educational programs and also by encouraging specialization in nursing services. This paralleled to some extent the evolution of medical specialties; as, for example, in providing for obstetrical, pediatric, and psychiatric nursing. Public health nursing, also, may be viewed as one of the specialties.

The need for psychiatric nursing became especially great, in view of the expansion of mental hospitals which came to include about half of all the institutional beds in the country. These hospitals were often isolated and it was not easy to persuade nurses to serve in them. They also presented a special problem, in that their need for men nurses in the male wards was imperative.

[55] Quoted in Esther Lucile Brown, *Nursing for the Future,* Russel Sage Foundation, New York, 1948, p. 80.

The early nursing schools, as noted, had largely limited their training to that of women. Between 1910 and 1940, the number of trained men nurses in the country rose slowly from 6,000 to 8,000; but their proportion to the total of graduate nurses fell from 7.4 to 2.3 per cent. In the mid-1940's, some seventy nursing schools possessed a few men students, but the total number of the latter was only 455. Four schools served men only.

This situation presented real difficulties. Even in some cases outside of mental hospitals, the service of men nurses was preferable to the usual combination of women nurses and orderlies; and the shortage of men became a chronic problem. The professional pendulum had swung a little too far in making nursing almost entirely a feminine vocation.

Developments in Nursing Education

As noted, the greater complexity of nursing services increased the pressure for improving the nursing schools. Most of them continued under hospital control and operated on a sub-professional level. Nursing organizations, hospital bodies, and foundations continued to conduct surveys and to make recommendations. Then, in 1941, came World War II, and with it some of the same phenomena observed during World War I. Women nurses (but not men) received commissions in the military services and this gave a further lift to their prestige. But after the War, in the later 1940's, the relative number of nursing students again declined.

This second "nursing shortage" could be ascribed to much the same trends as the first, but these had now gone further. It is true that real improvements in the working conditions of nursing had taken place during the 1930's and '40's. Nurses' homes had been made more comfortable, and the average weekly hours of duty had come down—along with those in other occupations—to about 45. In many hospitals, nurses were relieved of extreme formality and discipline, although adjustment to this new order of things was difficult for the older supervisors. And as medical care moved more and more into hospitals, there was less isolation in private duty in homes.

On the other hand, many new opportunities for women had emerged by this time in American society. Some of these paid better than did nursing, where salaries remained relatively low. And many vocations seemed to promise more freedom, if not actually a better future, than did that which opened out before the graduate nurse. In consequence, many potential nurses simply went into other fields.

The "nursing shortage" of recent years was a relative one in terms of demand; actually, there were more graduate nurses than there had ever been. Yet the situation was none the less serious. Hospitals, in seeking to overcome it, resorted to all sorts of ancillary services—to such volunteers as "grey ladies" on the one hand and to minimum-trained "ward helpers" or practical nurses on the other.

The most interesting aspect of the crisis in nursing, during the last two decades, was the manner in which it opened up debate on the whole place of nursing in American society and on the educational and other needs which were implicit in the situation. What types of nurses were needed and how should they be prepared?

These questions were especially pertinent because efforts to make nursing professional had made some headway by this time. In the first place, many good hospital schools at last decided to establish contacts with universities; and, by 1946, the number of these reached 91. In such schools, under a "five year plan," students could receive all the usual training and also secure a bachelor's degree. Although only a small percentage of those enrolled actually availed themselves of this opportunity, the arrangement seemed to have possibilities.

Going further, several universities—such as Minnesota and Yale—set up independent, professional schools of nursing, each with their own budgets and faculties. Such schools were analogous to those in business or engineering, in that they provided both general and vocational education in a four- or five-year curriculum.

The small number of nurses who received such professional education were qualified chiefly for teaching, for administration, or for specialized clinical services. What, then, of the need for personnel in the usual ward activities? The shortage of graduate nurses, in itself, raised again the possibility of recruiting what Dr. Mayo had once called "sub-nurses." And meantime, the very fact that graduate nurses were providing such complex services, likewise raised the question whether their more routine duties could not be handed over to less thoroughly trained people. Hence much interest was aroused in securing and training an adequate supply of practical nurses.

The desire to recruit this group was further heightened by the social repercussions of medical science. As preventive medicine and therapy grew more effective, life expectancy rose and the major disease problems became those of the chronic and degenerative diseases afflicting old age. A pressing need arose for more nursing homes (in the American sense) and for more chronic disease hospitals. In such institutions, as well as in homes, much of the nursing could be done on the practical level.

In response to this need, some hospitals set up practical-nurse training programs, and a few private schools did the same. More promising was the advent of training programs for practical nurses in public vocational schools maintained by boards of education. These provided at least several months of theoretical education, followed by work in the wards of a selected hospital. In some respects, recent programs for practical nurses were reminiscent of those provided for "trained nurses" in the early hospital schools.

There is no question about the need for practical nurses in homes and in certain types of institutions. As far as general hospitals are concerned, moreover, the hope is that they can take over the routine duties of graduate nurses and so combine with them in providing an effective ward team.

During World War II, it may be added, the Public Health Service organized a "Cadet Nursing Corps," and out of this grew arrangements for nursing education within Junior or "Community" Colleges. Under this program, students completed vocational training and also secured an "associate degree" at the end of two years. They were then, in some States, eligible to take the examinations required for graduate nurses. A report on these Junior College plans, prepared by Miss Mildred Montag of Teachers College, Columbia University, has been made available.

The solutions which may be found for the structural problems of nursing are not yet clear. Vocational levels in this field are particularly difficult to define: the professional nurse must apparently operate between physicians on the one hand and graduate nurses on the other. And the latter, in turn, find themselves in between professional personnel and practical nurses. There have been analogies to this situation in such fields as teaching and engineering, wherein all grades of preparation have been represented. More research on these matters in respect to nursing is needed, and it may be hoped that professional nurses will themselves contribute to studies of this nature.

Change in Structure of Nursing Organizations

Prospects for reaching conclusions about structural and professional matters in nursing improved, during recent decades, with the more effective organization of the field. It will be recalled that, after 1912, three major nursing societies were in existence—the American Nurses' Association (A.N.A.), the National League of Nursing Education (N.L.N.E.), and the National Organization of Public Health Nurses (N.O.P.H.N.). But as early as 1908, Martha Franklin—a graduate of the Woman's Hospital School in Philadelphia—had succeeded in organizing a National Association of Colored Graduate Nurses, which was eventually absorbed by the A.N.A. In later years, other special nursing societies were formed; notably the Association of Collegiate Schools of Nursing, the American Association of Industrial Nurses, and the National Association for Practical Nurse Education.

Meantime, an International Council of Nurses (I.C.N.) had been set up in 1900. This had been planned at an International Council of Women which had met at London the preceding year, and some of the same leaders were active here as had been involved in the planning of the N.L.N.E. at Chicago in 1893; notably, Mrs. Bedford Fenwick of the *British Journal of Nursing*, Mrs. Robb (Miss Hampton), and Miss Dock.

At the Berlin meeting of the I.C.N. in 1904, this body was organized to include one nursing society for each affiliated country; and the A.N.A. became the American constituent member. There were ten such national members by 1912, and eventually the number grew to thirty. The I.C.N., which now claims to be the largest association of professional women in the world, provided a forum for an international exchange of views which harmonized with the growing demand for international cooperation in all fields. In 1948 the I.C.N. established formal relations with the new World Health Organization of the United Nations.

On the home front, the American Nurses' Association was the largest and most representative body. It eventually developed a federated structure consistent with the American setting, which provided local and state units and a central body which included a council and house of delegates. The A.N.A. worked in close association with the National League for Nursing Education; and, as noted, the two societies jointly sponsored the *American Journal of Nursing.*

These organizational developments reflected the need for one major nursing association, and the parallel need—within that body— of a structure adapted to the size of the country. Some of the structure of the A.N.A., for example, was suggestive of that of the American Medical Association or of other bodies which worked out federated arrangements. Efforts were also made, within the A.N.A., to maintain a democratic representation in harmony with American political ideals.

At the same time, the appearance of seven other national nursing societies reflected the growth of specialized interests or of different types of training. As early as the 1920's, concern was expressed that the existence of these various bodies might weaken nursing by undermining its unity. The need for close cooperation among nursing groups was made more obvious by dissatisfaction, among individual nurses, with what seemed to them inadequate efforts to better the position of the guild. A few of them were inclined to turn away from all the nursing societies and to look rather to trade union affiliations as a source of support. Such a move was encouraged, at this time, by the interest which labor unions were themselves taking in industrial nursing. But a move to organize nurses' unions, whatever its advantages, would have been to abandon aspiration for future professional status. A similar dilemma confronted teachers in this same era.

Most nursing leaders, determined to maintain a guild rather than a labor tradition, sought to strengthen the field by closing its ranks. Consequently, proposals were made to merge some of the societies into one organization. But the difficulties facing such a merger were manifold; partially distinct fields and traditions, vested interests, and structural complications all stood in the way.

The problem was somewhat similar to that facing the many voluntary health societies (the National Tuberculosis Association, the American Heart Association, et cetera), wherein there was much talk of mergers in the 1920's and again in the '40's. In that field, a single National Health Council was set up—with which the A.N.A. was affiliated—but this body did not become more than a coordinating and consultative one.

In the nursing field, in contrast, the unification program was carried much farther. A series of conferences, begun before World War II but carried to completion during post-war years, laid the plans for merging certain societies. This effort involved studies of structure, a high degree of cooperation, and an expenditure of funds raised by the nursing societies themselves.

It was therefore greatly to the credit of the groups involved that finally, in 1952, the National League for Nursing Education, the National Organization of Public Health Nurses, and the Association of Collegiate Schools of Nursing were merged into the National League for Nursing. This body, which combines the major, special programs in nursing education, was set up in harmony with the general membership group (A.N.A.); and these two associations coordinated and spoke for the nursing field as a whole.

Professional Status of Nursing

Nursing is still, in the mid-twentieth century, a field in flux. The complexity of its problems is only matched by the value of its achievements. If one looks only at these achievements, it is easy to present the whole story of nursing as one of remarkable progress, especially over the period of the last seventy-five years. If, on the other hand, one focuses entirely on present difficulties, more critical comments are in order. Historical perspectives, at this point, may help in striking a balance between extremes in attitudes.

Several facts are clear. In the first place, there is no question that nursing on the upper levels has been greatly improved during recent generations. In no country has this been more obvious than in the United States. This trend resulted in part from the efforts of devoted women, who were moved originally by the same humanitarianism which had inspired nursing throughout the ages. But the women who led nursing programs after 1870 realized that better nursing was also demanded by a new type of medical science; and in blending humane with scientific goals, they enabled nursing to adjust to medicine and so to serve the needs of modern societies for medical care.

This process was not an easy one. It was retarded at many points by medical skepticism, by the vested interests of hospitals, and by the limitations of a social tradition which had long placed nursing little above the servant level. The extent to which the upper levels of nursing can attain to full professional status is not clear even today.

Yet it is here that the historical perspective can be of service. There is no doubt that nursing has been moving *toward* professional status, and that it may move further in the future. Only contrast the position and prospects of nursing in the 1950's, with those which faced the pioneer nurses of 1873! In that earlier day, earnest but unorganized women stood almost alone in initiating the first efforts to train lay women as nurses. Today, large and well organized bodies, including the hospitals, public schools, universities, foundations, and government agencies as well as the nursing associations, are vitally concerned with the improvement of nursing as a whole.

One other thing may be learned from the leaders of 1873. Their vision of service to mankind can be and should be as meaningful today as it was in that earlier time. Lay nurses have the same right as do those in other vocations to be concerned about adequate income and working conditions, but it would be an unhappy outcome if nurses were to limit their outlook to these considerations. Society expects that nurses, like teachers, physicians, and clergymen, will be animated also by a desire to serve. If this spirit is maintained, nursing will continue to be a calling as well as a vocation; and the rewards of a calling transcend those of a trade.

To put this in another way, the needs of suffering humanity are still as real, in this age of scientific medicine, as they were in the Middle Ages. And those who minister to these needs with all the latest techniques, merit much of the respect which was accorded those Sisters of a bygone age who served without benefit of bacteriology or chemotherapy.

Hence nursing may go forward in terms of both its humane and its scientific traditions. Well prepared and competent nurses are essential to modern society. Without them the hospitals would close. And in the humane tradition, their opportunities and services mav well be greater than those of physicians themselves.

Florence Nightingale realized this, and the realization imparted to all her activities a dignity which was acknowledged throughout the world. Her followers in the United States adjusted her ideals to the realities of the American scene, among which were those of evolving medical achievement. We now recognize that neither science nor humanitarianism is, in itself, enough. But nursing which is both scientific *and* humane can confront the future with confidence.

Index

Aesculapius, 41
Agriculture, scientific, 177
Aikenhead, Mary, 269
Alexandria, origin of medical research in, 61
All Saints Sisterhood, 270
Almshouses, 155, 172, 288
America, development of hospitals in, 170
  development of nursing in, 170
  English in, 172
  French in, 171
  Spanish in, 170
American Association of Industrial Nurses, 315
American Red Cross, founding of, 308
American Society of Superintendents of Training Schools for Nurses of the United States and Canada, 304
American Hospital Association, 306
American Journal of Nursing, 305, 316
American Nurses' Association, 305, 315
Anatomy, in eighteenth century, 195
  in nineteenth century, 252
  Renaissance, 137
Anesthesia, discovery of, 255
  in late Middle Ages, 101
  in nineteenth century, 256
Angles, conquest of Britain by, 86
Anglicans, 172
Anglican Church, hospitals and, 159
Anglican Sisters, improvement of hospital training by, 271
Anthropologists, primitive cultures discovered by, 3

Antisepsis, discovery of, 258
Apothecaries, practice of medicine by, 212
Apothecaries Guild, 147
Arabs, influence of, on Europe, 94
Archeologists, evidence of primitive medicine uncovered by, 3
Archimedes, physics and, 71
Architecture, Renaissance, 121
Aristotle, 46, 94
Army Nursing Corps, beginnings of, 308
Art, development of, in Renaissance, 117
  in eighteenth century, 186
Artisans, Renaissance, 129
Asceticism, Christian, 80
Asepsis, employment during late Middle Ages, 102
Association of Collegiate Schools of Nursing, 315
Astrology, influence on primitive medicine, 1
Athens, as center of Greek civilization, 40
Augsburg Confession, 126
Augustinian Sisters, 162, 167
  in Canada, 171

Babylonia, legal codes of, 29
  medicine and surgery in, 29
Bacon, Roger, 95
Banting, Frederick, 262
Baptists, 126

319